医療従事者のための
医学英語入門

清水雅子／著

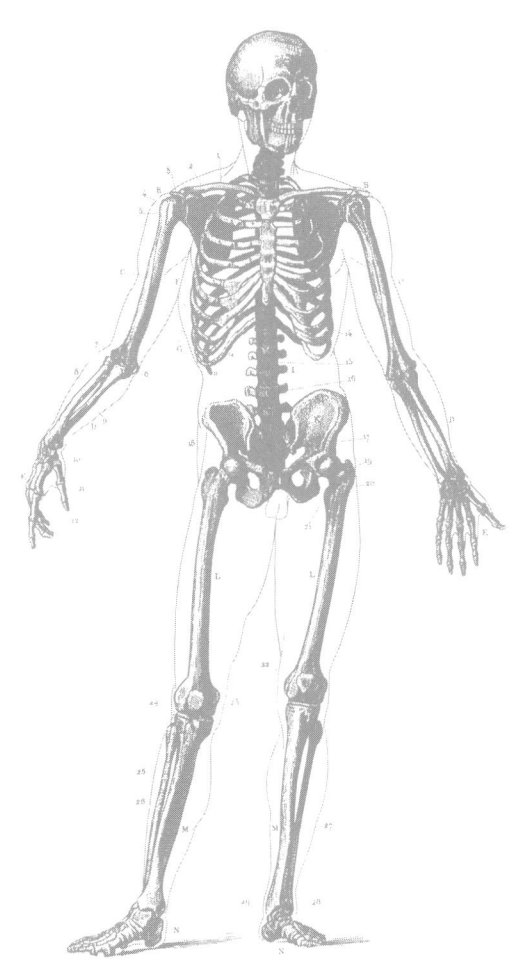

講談社

出 典 一 覧

A　*THE HUMAN BODY*
　　Edward P. Ortleb and Richard Cadice
　　Milliken Publishing Company ©1986

B　*The World Book Encyclopedia* Vol. 2, 6, 8, 12, 16.
　　World Book, Inc. ©1988

C　*Diseases of the Human Body 4th edition*
　　Carol D. Tamparo and Marci A. Lewis
　　F. A. Davis Company ©2005

D　*The Sea and Poison*（Shusaku Endo）
　　A Novel translated from the Japanese by Michael Gallanger ©1972
　　Peter Owen, London

E　Wikipedia, "2009 flu pandemic"
　　http://en.wikipedia.org/wiki/2009_flu_pandemic

F　Wikipedia, "Organ transplantation"
　　http://en.wikipedia.org/wiki/Organ_transplantation

G　日本臓器移植ネットワークホームページ
　　http://www.jotnw.or.jp/english/index.html

H　Wikipedia, "Skin"
　　http://en.wikipedia.org/wiki/Skin

I　Wikipedia, "Human nose"
　　http://en.wikipedia.org/wiki/Human_nose

J　Wikipedia, "Tongue"
　　http://en.wikipedia.org/wiki/Tongue

K　*The Doctor's Wife*（Sawako Ariyoshi）
　　Translated by Wakako Hironaka and Ann Kostant ©1978
　　Kodansha International, Tokyo

L　*The Symposium*（Plato）
　　Translated by Walter Hamilton ©1951
　　Penguin Books, England

M　『楢山節考』
　　深沢七郎著，©1964
　　新潮社

まえがき

　本書は，拙著『医療技術者のための医学英語入門』（1991）を，新版『医療従事者のための医学英語入門』として改訂したものです．

　旧版の出版後，20年の間に世の中は著しく変貌し，とりわけ医療・医学分野における変化・発展には目覚ましいものがあります．この度の改訂では，旧著の構成と内容を全般的に見直し，可能な限り修正を加えました．具体的には，情報としてすでに古くなった題材を除き，アップトゥーデートな話題を取り入れました．もちろん，医学・医療領域の基本は身体であり，医学英語の基準は身体用語にあることに変わりはありません．したがって，基本的には旧版同様に，各器官・組織の構造・機能を中心とし，平易で簡潔な英文を選びました．また，医学英語の原則的な特徴については，10項目からなるコラム「医学英語の常識」の中で解説しました．

　専門領域の英語学習は，とかく単調になり，その難解さに挫折しがちです．学習に興味をもち，楽しく継続していくために，「医学英語のルーツ—ギリシア神話」というコラムを設けました．一見無関係と思われる神話の世界に，医学英語のルーツが潜んでいることに着目したものです．取り上げたトピックスは，筆者がこれまで授業で紹介し，学生たちが興味を示したものから選びました．同時に，文学作品等から，4篇の英訳文の抜粋を選んでいます．本書を手にされた方々が，これをきっかけに，実用的な英語のみならず，人間性への洞察を深め，優れたコミュニケーション能力を身につけた医療の専門家を目指されるよう願っております．

　偶々，旧版を目にされた講談社サイエンティフィクの編集者，三浦洋一郎氏から，「是非，このようなテキスト作成に携わってみたい」とのお話をいただき，改訂新版が実現しました．さらに，作業の過程でも，さまざまな視点から貴重

なご助言をいただきました．心より感謝申し上げます．

2011 年 2 月

清水　雅子

初 版 ま え が き

　本書は，高等学校を卒業し，初めて医学英語に接する医学・医療技術系の学生を対象に書かれたものです．医学・医療の基本である人体の主要な組織を中心に記述しておりますが，初心者が親しみやすいようにと，各組織や器官についての説明文はできるだけ簡潔で，平易な英語で書かれたものを選びました．一方，多様な英文に接することも重要であると考え，さまざまな文献からの引用を心掛け，なじみのうすい英単語，とくに医学用語については邦語訳を付しました．

　筆者は，この十年間，川崎医科大学，川崎医療短期大学教養課程における英語教育に携わってまいりましたが，専門課程への橋渡しとなる医学英語を手ほどきすることの重要性を痛感すると同時に，さらに将来医学・医療に従事する学生達に広い視野をもった人間観を育んでほしいと常々願っておりました．本書のReadingおよびコラムの欄は，こういった意図の下に，教材あるいはトピックスとして選んだものです．しかしいずれの英文も古物全体からの部分的な抜粋にすぎません．このテキストの読み物をきっかけにして，是非自分で一冊二冊と読み進め，そこに描かれた人間への温かい思いや深い愛情に感動をおぼえ，医学における人間性の問題を考えることによって，秀れたスペシャリストになってほしいと願っております．もちろん，世界のさまざまな人々とのコミュニケイションに役立つ英語そのものへの理解・関心を一層深めることも心掛けてほしいと思います．

　本書の執筆にあたり数々の貴重なご教示を賜りました川崎医科大学名誉教授中川定明先生，ならびに出版への仲介の労をおとりくださり，数々の貴重なご助言を賜りました川崎医療福祉大学教授梶谷文彦先生に心から感謝申し上げます．なお，講談社サイエンティフィク吉田茂子部長には，立案から校正に至るまで

大変お世話になりました．心からお礼申し上げます．

1990 年 12 月

著者

目　次

まえがき ...... *iii*
初版まえがき ...... *v*

CHAPTER 1　The Human Body　人体 1
　What is the body made up of?　身体は何から構成されているか？
　Cell — 細胞
　Tissue, organ and system — 組織，器官，体系
　Characteristics of the human body　人体の特徴
　医学英語の常識（1）　薬指は medical finger ?　身体の英語と日本語のズレにご用心

CHAPTER 2　The Skeletal System　骨格系 10
　Background Information
　The constitution of the human skeleton（main bones）　骨格の構成
　Joint（articulation）— 関節
　医学英語の常識（2）　医学英語の基本 3 項
　医学英語のルーツ — ギリシア神話（1）　atlas（環椎）は Atlas（アトラス）から

CHAPTER 3　The Muscular System　筋肉系 24
　Background Information
　Tendon — 腱
　Ligament — 靭帯

Movement — 運動
医学英語の常識（3）　医学英語の構成
医学英語のルーツ — ギリシア神話（2）　踵（かかと）の腱は，ギリシア神話の英雄アキレウスのアキレス腱

CHAPTER 4　The Circulatory System　循環系　…… 35
Background Information
The constitution of the blood　血液の成分
Heart — 心臓
Background Information
医学英語の常識（4）　複数形
医学英語のルーツ — ギリシア神話（3）　その一言が…？　英雄ペルセウスと「メドゥーサの頭」(Medusa head)

CHAPTER 5　The Lymphatic System　リンパ系　…… 47
Background Information
Parts of the lymphatic system — リンパ系の部位
Spleen — 脾臓
Treatment of cancer　癌の治療
　（1）Surgery — 外科手術
　（2）Radiation therapy — 放射線療法
　（3）Chemotherapy — 化学療法
　（4）Immunotherapy（Biotherapy）— 免疫療法（生物学的療法）
　（5）Hormonal therapy — ホルモン療法
　（6）Alternative therapy — 代替療法
医学英語の常識（5）　語源と医学英語：cancer（癌）はなぜ蟹？
医学英語のルーツ — ギリシア神話（4）　モルヒネは眠りの神ヒュピノスの息子モルペウスから，麻薬中毒は自己愛者ナルキッソスから

CHAPTER 6　　The Respiratory System　　呼吸器系　　　　…… 62
　　Background Information
　　Alveoli and other respiratory tubes ― 肺胞と呼吸器官
　　Supplementary Reading　　The Sea and Poison（海と毒薬）
　　医学英語の常識（6）　新型インフルエンザ

CHAPTER 7　　The Digestive System　　消化器系　　　　…… 74
　　The main digestive organs　主要消化器官
　　　（1）Teeth and salivary glands ― 歯，唾液腺
　　　（2）Esophagus and the stomach ― 食道と胃
　　　（3）Small intestine ― 小腸
　　　（4）Large intestine ― 大腸
　　The accessory digestive organs　付属消化器官
　　Liver and gallbladder ― 肝臓・胆のう
　　医学英語の常識（7）　病名と冠詞
　　医学英語のルーツ ― ギリシア神話（5）　接頭辞 epi- と pro- とプロメテウスの肝臓，そして pan- とパンドーラ

CHAPTER 8　　The Urinary System　　泌尿器系　　　　…… 89
　　Background Information
　　Nephron ― ネフロン（腎単位）
　　医学英語の常識（8）　略語，略語，略語

CHAPTER 9　　The Nervous System　　神経系　　　　…… 98
　　Background Information
　　Spinal cord ― 脊髄
　　Brain ― 脳
　　Background Information
　　The work of the brain ― 脳の働き
　　The work of the brain: in the use of language ― 言語の使用における脳の働き

Brain death and Organ transplantation　脳死と臓器移植
医学英語のルーツ ― ギリシア神話（6）　蜘蛛とクモ膜とアラクネ

CHAPTER 10　The Sense Organs　感覚器官　……116
Eye ― 目
Focusing ― 焦点調節
Ear ― 耳
Skin ― 皮膚
Nose ― 鼻
Tongue ― 舌
Supplementary Reading　The Doctor's Wife（華岡青洲の妻）
医学英語のルーツ ― ギリシア神話（7）　心の目：知らずして父を殺し，母と結婚した息子，オイディプス

CHAPTER 11　Endocrine/Exocrine System
　　　　　　　内分泌系，外分泌系　……132
Endocrine glands ― 内分泌腺
Exocrine glands ― 外分泌腺
Glandlike structures ― 腺様構造
Medical uses of hormones ― ホルモン療法
医学英語の常識（9）　医学に貢献する fruit fly

CHAPTER 12　The Reproductive System　生殖系　……142
Background Information
Human reproduction ― ヒトの生殖
　（1）The male reproductive system ― 男性の生殖系
　（2）The female reproductive system ― 女性の生殖系
Supplementary Reading　Symposium（饗宴：アリストファネスのことば）
医学英語のルーツ ― ギリシア神話（8）　Love（愛）= Psyche（プシュケ）+ Eros（エロス）

CHAPTER 13　Aging and the end of life　加齢と生の終焉　……154
 Aging ― 加齢
 Death ― 死
  (1) Medical aspects of death ― 死の医学的側面
  (2) Defining death ― 死の定義
  (3) The right to die ― 死ぬ権利
 医学英語の常識 (10)　What is human？― 語源から導かれること
 Supplementary Reading　Consideration on NARAYAMA Song（楢山節考）
 医学英語のルーツ ― ギリシア神話 (9)　Man is mortal ― 永遠の眠りの神タナトス（Tanatos）を受容するということ

Appendix　……171
 Terms for hospital（病院用語）
 Names of diseases（病名）
 Symptom（病気の兆候）
 Expression of wound, etc.（傷の表現）
 Types of medicine（薬の種類）
 Terms of examination（検査用語）
 Common medical abbreviations（略語）
 Prefix（接頭辞）
 Suffix（疾患とかかわる接尾辞）
 Combining forms and medical terms（連結形）

CHAPTER 1
The Human Body 人体

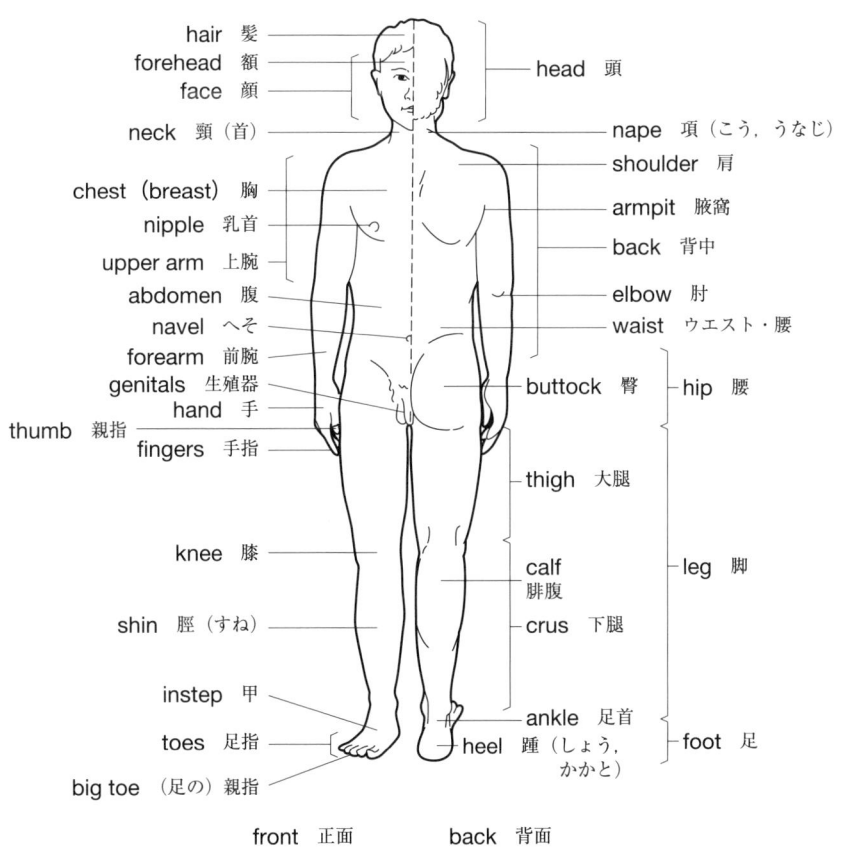

front 正面　　back 背面

The Human Body

Have you ever asked yourself any questions like these — How do I stand erect and tall?　How do I move?　How do I do such simple, taken-for-granted things as washing my face, or brushing my teeth, or combing my hair?　And how do diseases as different as poliomyelitis, strokes, and arthritis make me unable to move normally?　If I touch something, how do I know that I have touched it and how do I detect whether it is hot or cold, smooth or rough, wet or dry?　How do I see?　Hear?　Taste?　Smell?　Why must I eat and breathe to live?　Why must my heart beat?　Answers to these and many more questions can be found within the pages of this book.

What is the body made up of?
身体は何から構成されているか？

Just as any building is made up of many kinds of structural units (walls, floors, steel, glass, bricks, nails, for instance), so too the body is made up of different kinds of structural units.

Here, listed in order from the smallest and simplest to the largest and most complex, are the names of the body's structural units: cells, tissues, organs, and systems.

Cell — 細胞

About three hundred years ago, Robert Hooke looked through his microscope (one of the very early ones) at some plant material.　What he saw must have surprised him.　Instead of a single, much enlarged piece of plant material, he saw a group of many small pieces. They looked like miniature prison cells to him, so that is what he called them — cells. Hooke's discovery that plants were made up of cells proved to be a foundation stone for modern biology. Thousands of individuals have examined thousands of plant and animal specimens since Hooke's time and have found all of them made up of cells. Today, therefore, biologists think of a cell as the unit of structure of living things, just as you might think of a brick as the unit of structure of a brick wall or of a brick house.

When a living thing is made up of a great many cells, its cells are not all alike. They differ somewhat in structure. Also, because structure determines function, they differ in certain functions. Cells with one type of structure, for example, conduct impulses; cells with a different type of structure contract; cells with still another type of structure secrete, and so on. Four main types of cells compose our bodies; epithelial cells, connective cells, muscle cells, and nerve cells.

Tissue, organ and system — 組織，器官，体系

A *tissue* is a group of similar cells with varying amounts and kinds of material filling in any spaces between the cells. Although there are only four main kinds of tissues — epithelial, connective, muscular, and nervous — there are many subtypes.

An *organ* is a structure composed of several kinds of tissues — often of all four main kinds. ... Organs perform more complex functions for the body than any single cell or single tissue can perform alone.

The Human Body

You probably already know the names of most of the organs—stomach, intestines, liver, gallbladder, heart, lungs, eyes, ears, and many others.

胃〔stʌ́mək〕, 腸, 肝臓〔lívər〕, 胆のう, 心臓, 肺

A *system* is the largest structural unit in the body. It consists of a group of organs that work together to perform a more complex function than any one organ can perform alone. Most anatomists group organs into the following nine systems; skeletal, muscular, circulatory, digestive, respiratory, urinary, reproductive, endocrine, and nervous.

解剖学者

骨格, 筋, 循環, 消化, 呼吸, 泌尿, 生殖, 内分泌, 神経 (系)

What structures make up the body? Briefly, cells, tissues, organs, and systems. Millions of similar cells form each tissue, two or more kinds of tissues form each organ, several organs form each system, and nine systems form the body.

Let's pronounce medical English terms.

1. epitherial cell 2. muscular tissue 3. microscope
4. stomach

Review questions

1. What did Robert Hooke find through his simple microscope about 300 years ago?
2. Why do all cells differ in their functions?
3. What structures make up the body?
4. Select the appropriate definition for each word.
    1) cell   (   )
    2) tissue   (   )
    3) organ   (   )
    4) system   (   )
    5) structure (   )
        a. a structure that are formed by millions of cells

Tissue, organ and system

b. a part of the body that has an independent form, such as the stomach or the lung
c. a set of organs in the body with a common structure or function
d. the smallest unit of living matter that can exist on its own
e. a set of arrangement of the human body that are connected together

The Human Body

Characteristics of the human body
人体の特徴

Human beings and the other primates share many physical features. For example, both human beings and apes rely on their excellent vision for much of their information about the environment. They have large eyes, sensitive retinas, and *stereoscopic vision* (the ability to perceive depth). Human beings and apes also have a highly developed nervous system and a large brain. Human beings and many other primates have long, flexible fingers and *opposable thumbs,* which can be placed opposite the fingers for grasping. In addition, their fingers and toes have nails instead of claws.

霊長類
特徴
サル

網膜，視野

柔軟な指，(他の指と)向い合わせになる親指

Many of the physical characteristics that distinguish human beings from other primates are related to the ability of people to stand upright and walk on two legs. This ability chiefly requires long, powerful legs. The human rump has strong muscles that propel the body forward and balance the trunk alternately on each leg when a person walks. In contrast, apes spend most of their time climbing and swinging in trees or walking on all four limbs. Their rumps have relatively weak muscles, and their arms are longer and stronger than their legs.

臀部，筋肉〔mʌsl〕
胴体

四肢

The human spine, unlike the spine of any other animal, has a curve in the lower back. This curve helps make upright posture possible by placing the body's center of gravity directly over the pelvis. The human foot is also specially adapted for walking on two legs. Apes use all four limbs to support their weight, and

脊柱〔spaɪn〕

立位
重力，骨盤

they can grasp objects almost as well with their feet as with their hands. In human beings, however, the feet support the entire weight of the body, and the toes have little ability to grasp or to move independently.

The human brain is extremely well developed and at least twice as large as any ape's brain. Because of the brain's size, the human skull is rounder than any other primate's skull.　頭蓋骨

Let's pronounce medical English terms.

1. retina　　2. vision　　3. limb　　4. spine
5. pelvis　　6. muscle（綴り注意）　　7. brain

Review questions

1. Select the characteristics of human beings, which are different from the other primates.
    a. excellent vision
    b. underdeveloped nervous system
    c. opposable thumbs
    d. upright standing position
    e. straight spine
    f. extremely developed brain
    g. weak muscle of the rump

The Human Body

医学英語の常識（1）
薬指は medical finger？　身体の英語と日本語のズレにご用心

　英語では手の指を finger，足の指を toe とよぶ．We have five fingers on each hand. とまとめていい，また親指を特別に扱い，We have a thumb and four fingers. ともいう[1]．足の親指は big toe，ほかの指は toe と素っ気ないが，手の指には以下の図のようにそれぞれ個別に名称が与えられている．それは，人間の豊かな生活と文化の発展が，手と手指なくしてあり得なかったことを表わしているのであろう．

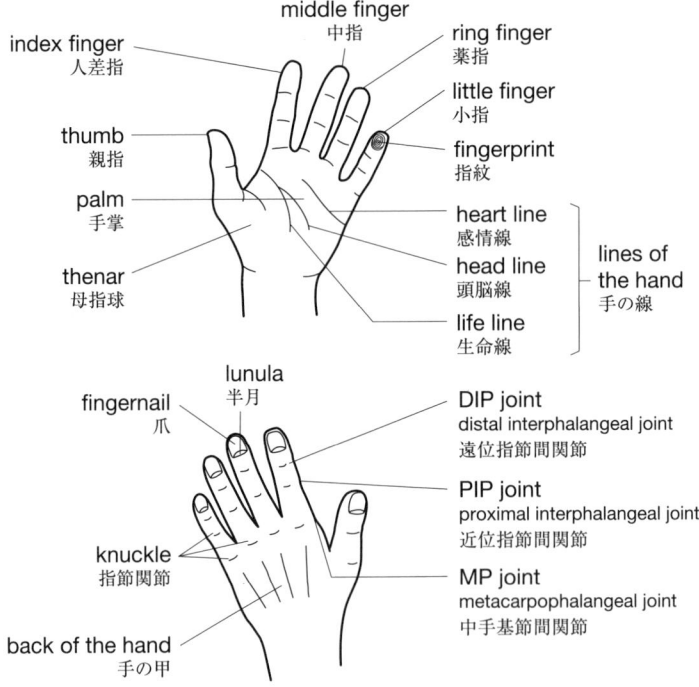

　注）定冠詞 the を省略．また，各指は隠れた意味をもつので動作には要注意である．

　とくに thumb[2] は，ほかの指のように〜finger とはよばれず特別視されているが，これは，親指の母指対向性（opposable thumb）が人間に多くのこ

とを可能にしてきたという理由が背後にある．

ほかにも日英対称でない第3指がある．「薬指」はかつて薬を溶かすのに使ったことから，ring finger は結婚指輪をはめることから命名されている．それでは，英語に medical finger はあるだろうか．世界に冠たる *OED*（*Oxford English Dictionary*，全20巻）の finger の項には，ring finger（annular, †leech-, †medical, †physic-finger）と記述されており，英語にも medical finger がある．しかし，記号の † が obsolete word（廃語）という意味であるため，現在，medical finger は過去の言葉である．

このように身体の器官を表わす日英語の表現のズレに注意しよう．以下にいくつかの例をあげる．

例1）日本語の"腰"は英語では次の部分である．

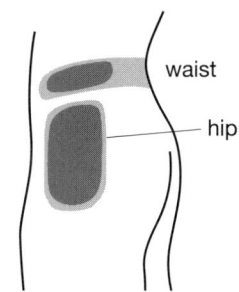

例2）face：head の一部．顔：顔の全部分．
例3）throat：首の前面，咽喉．日本語：首の前部．

注
1) 最近では親指を the first finger とし，順に，second, third, 薬指を the fourth finger とする解剖学書が多い．
2) この語は古期英語（1150年ごろ以前の英語）では thūma（膨張の意味）であったが，13世紀末に b が添字されて thumb となった．

CHAPTER 2
The Skeletal System　骨格系

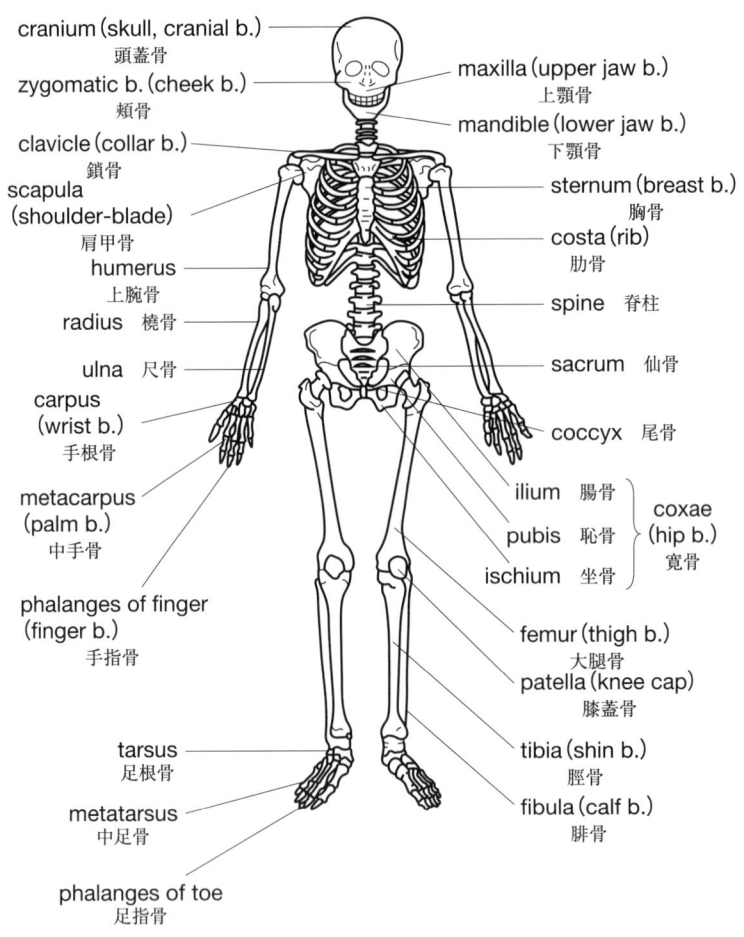

Background Information

The skeletal system of the human body consists of 206-210 bones. Some small bones in the feet and hands vary in number from person to person.

Bone is a dry, dense tissue composed of a calcium-phosphorus mineral (65%), and organic matter and water (35%). Bone is covered with a living membrane called the periosteum which contains bone-forming cells, the osteoblasts. During embryonic development, the skeletal framework is composed of cartilage and membranes. The osteoblasts replace the cartilage and membranes with bony tissue. The center of bone contains marrow in which are found blood vessels, fat cells, and some blood forming tissue. There are four main shapes of bone. Ribs are examples of flat bones. Vertebrae are examples of irregular shaped bones. Wrist and ankle bones are examples of short bones. The humerus bone of the arm and the femur bone of the leg are examples of long bones.

The skeletal system is usually divided into the axial skeleton and the appendicular skeleton. The axial skeleton consists of the skull, spinal column (made up of 33 vertebrae) and the ribs (12 pairs). The appendicular skeleton consists of the bones of the shoulder and arms and those of the pelvis and legs. Healthy bones combine strength and weight-bearing ability with lightness in weight.

リン酸カルシウム

骨膜

骨芽細胞, 胎児の発達

軟骨

髄

脊椎

軸骨格
体肢骨格

〔出典 A, p.ii：L6～L31〕

The Skeletal System

The constitution of the human skeleton（main bones）骨格の構成

1）Axial skeleton　軸骨格（80）
　　cranium　頭蓋（22）
　　　　neurocranium　脳頭蓋（8）
　　　　viscerocranium　顔面頭蓋（14）
　　appendicular bones of cranium　付属骨（7）
　　　　auditory ossicles　耳小骨（6）
　　　　hyoid bone　舌骨（1）
　　thorax　胸郭（25）
　　　　sternum　胸骨（1）
　　　　costa　肋骨（24）
　　spine　脊柱（26）
　　　　vertebra　脊椎（複数形 vertebrae）（24）
　　　　sacrum　仙骨（1）
　　　　coccyx　尾骨（1）

2）Appendicular skeleton　体肢骨格（126）
　　＊pectoral girdle　上肢帯（4）
　　　　clavicle　鎖骨（2）
　　　　scapula　肩甲骨（2）
　　＊upper limbs　上肢（60）
　　　　humerus　上腕骨（2）
　　　　radius　橈骨（2）
　　　　ulna　尺骨（2）
　　　　carpus　手根骨（16）
　　　　metacarpus　中手骨（10）
　　　　phalanx（複数形 phalanges）　手指骨（28）
　　＊pelvic girdle　下肢帯（2）
　　　　hip bone　寛骨（2）
　　＊lower limbs　下肢（60）
　　　　femur　大腿骨（2）
　　　　patella　膝蓋骨（2）
　　　　tibia　脛骨（2）
　　　　fibula　腓骨（2）
　　　　tarsal bone　足根骨（14）
　　　　metatarsal bone　中足骨（10）
　　　　phalanx（複数形 phalanges）　趾節骨（28）

注
1）（　）の中の数字は椎骨の数を表す．
2）リストの名称は TA（Terminologia anatomica 国際解剖学用語）に基づく．TA

については後述.
3) sacrum（1）は，sacral vertebrae 仙椎 5 椎が癒合.
4) coccyx（1）は，coccygeal vertebrae 尾椎 2〜4 椎が癒合.
5) hip bone（3）は，ilium（腸骨），ischium（坐骨），pubis（恥骨）が癒合.
6) 複数形については，ラテン語独特の形があるが，ここでは vertebra/vertebrae と phalynx/phalynges にとどめた．そのほかのルールについては, p.43 を参照.

Spine　脊柱

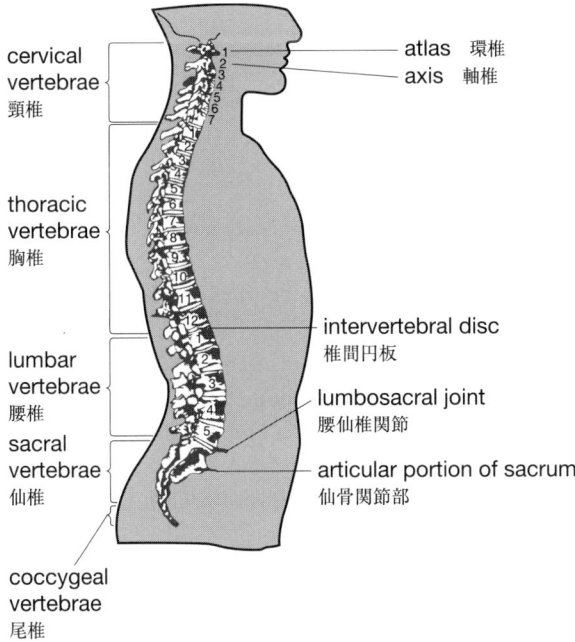

The Skeletal System

The bone structure (long bone) 骨の構造（長骨）

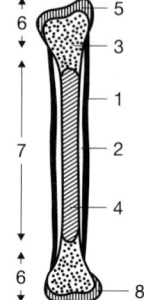

1. periosteum 骨膜
2. compact bone 緻密質
3. cancellous bone 海綿質
4. medullary cavity 骨髄腔
5. articular cartilage 関節軟骨
6. epiphysis 骨端
7. diaphysis 骨幹
8. joint capsule 関節包

Let's pronounce medical English terms.

1. skeleton (綴り注意)　2. limb　3. vertebrae
4. cartilage　5. cranium　6. clavicle

Review questions

1. How many bones does the human body have?
2. What tissues is the bone composed of?
3. What organ is the axial skeleton and the appendicular one composed of?
4. Write the English name of parts of the bone for each phrase.
   1) living membrane around the bone (　　　)
   2) the center of the bone in which blood cells are produced (　　　)
   3) hard outer surface of the bone (　　　)
5. Select the appropriate medical English for each word.
   1) collarbone　　　(　　)
   2) shoulder blade　(　　)
   3) skull　　　　　(　　)
   4) shinbone　　　 (　　)
   5) rib　　　　　　(　　)
   a. cranium　　b. costa　　c. tibia
   d. clavicle　　e. scapula

Joint (articulation) — 関節

Joint is the place at which two or more bones meet in the skeleton of the body. This place is also called an *articulation*. Joints may be *fixed* or *movable*. Fixed joints are seams between bones that lie directly against each other, or are separated only by a thin layer of connective tissue. In case of a blow or an accident, these joints may absorb just enough shock to keep the bones from breaking. The joints of the cranium (covering of the brain) are fixed and protect the brain.

There are three main kinds of movable joints: (1) *hinge* joints, (2) *pivot* joints, and (3) *ball-and-socket* joints. Hinge joints are those that permit a forward and backward motion in one plane, like the motion of a door on its hinges. The joints at the knee and fingers are modified hinge joints. Pivot joints give a rotating motion, such as the movement of the head from side to side. The elbow has both hinge and pivot joints. Ball-and-socket joints allow the greatest freedom of movement. These joints are made up of a large round end of a long bone that fits into the hollow of another bone. The hip and shoulder have ball-and-socket joints. The arms of the body can move more freely than the legs because of the way that the joints are arranged, and because the shoulder blade is only loosely attached to the chest wall.

Movable joints are protected from wear and tear in several ways. A smooth layer of *cartilage* (gristle) covers the ends of bones that move over one another. The elasticity of cartilage breaks the force of sudden shocks. Also, the smooth quality of the cartilage

The Skeletal System

makes a joint move easily. A liquid called *synovial fluid* keeps the joints moist and lubricated.   滑液

Bones are held together at the joint by strong ligaments that attach above and below the joint. At the hip, a number of ligaments circle the bone like a collar to keep the joint in place.   …をとりまく / …を適所に保つ

Joints are often sprained or dislocated. A sprain occurs when the ligaments around a joint are torn or badly stretched. Serious sprains are painful, and if neglected may result in instability of the joint. Dislocated joints should be treated as soon as possible by a physician. Inflammation of the joints may result from infections or from such disorders as arthritis.   捻挫する, 脱臼する / 不安定 / 炎症 / 感染, 疾患

Shoulder　肩

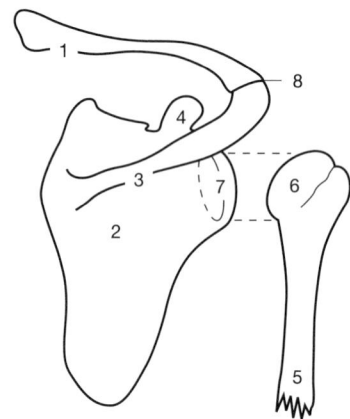

1. clavicle　鎖骨　　　　　　　2. scapula　肩甲骨
3. spine　脊柱
4. coracoid process　烏口突起(coraco-＝烏, process＝突起)
5. humerus　上腕骨　　　　　　6. head of humerus　上腕骨頭
7. glenoid cavity　関節窩(gleno-＝ソケット)　8. acromion　肩峰(acro-＝先端)

Joint (articulation)

Knee　膝

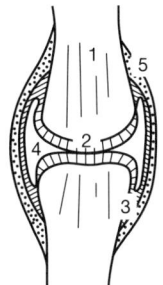

1. bone　骨
2. articular cartilage　関節性軟骨
3. synovial membrane　滑膜
4. synovial cavity and fluid　滑膜腔／滑膜液
5. joint capsule　関節包（骨端を包む袋状構造，外層：結合組織．内層：滑膜．）

Let's pronounce medical English terms.

1. arthritis　　2. articulation　　3. ligament
4. inflammation　　5. sprain

Review questions

1. Give the names of movable joints and explain each function briefly.
2. Tell the functions of the cartilage in brief.
3. Select the appropriate Japanese for each word.
   1) arthritis　　(　　)
   2) cartilage　　(　　)
   3) joint　　(　　)
   4) ligament　　(　　)
   5) sprain　　(　　)
   a. 捻挫　b. 靭帯　c. 関節　d. 軟骨　e. 関節炎
4. Write the plural forms of each word below.
   a. cranium　　(　　)
   b. scapula　　(　　)
   c. humerus　　(　　)
   d. coccyx　　(　　)

The Skeletal System

5. Write the English terms for each joint below according to the English sentences.

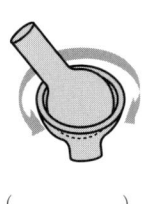   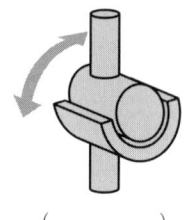   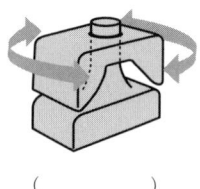

(   )   (   )   (   )

〔参考〕上記以外の関節

(1) movable joints　可動関節

plane joint　平面(滑動)関節　　condylar joint　楕円関節　　saddle joint　鞍関節

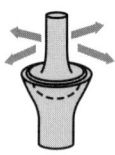   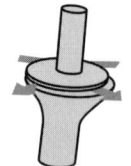   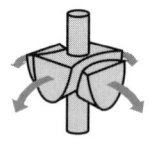

例：手や足の屈曲運動　　例：手首の前後の屈曲運動および内，外回りの回転運動　　例：親指の回転運動．但し一定範囲の回転

(2) fixed joints　固定関節

　　　脛骨と腓骨の接点　　　　　　頭蓋骨は，骨が結合して縫合(suture)を形成する

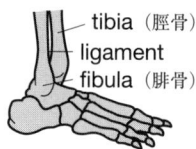   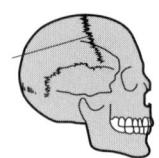

tibia（脛骨）
ligament
fibula（腓骨）

医学英語の常識（2）
医学英語の基本3項

　医学英語って面倒！　とすでに諦めている人はいませんか？　Practice makes perfect.（習うより慣れろ）です．けれども，闇雲に突き進んでも効果が低いので，最初に医学英語の常識ともいえる特徴を3つ挙げておこう．

1. TA（Terminologia Anatomica：国際解剖学用語）について
　このテキストの1章が骨格系，筋肉系ではじまる理由は，身体が医学の基礎であり，医学英語の基準が解剖学用語にあるからだ．解剖学用語は19世紀に至るまで国と地域によって異なっていた．IFAA（国際解剖学会連合）が1903年以来，解剖学の概念と用語の標準化に取り組み，長い時間をかけて協議・改訂し，1997年正式に公表された．その数，約7500語．しかし，用語集には公式用語のラテン語に加えて，国際社会において医学・科学の意思疎通に必要な英語が付加された．たとえば，寛骨はラテン語の os coxae に加えて，coxal bone，英語の hip bone も TA．医学英語は必ずしもラテン語だけではない，と知っておこう．

2. TAが基本的にラテン語である理由について
　医学英語に特にギリシア語・ラテン語由来の用語が多いのは，医学が，かの医学の祖と敬われるギリシアのヒポクラテス（Hippocrates）が実践した"臨床（bedside）で観察（observation）・記録（recording）"に倣いラテン語が学問用語であった間に体系を形成してきた歴史をもつからだ．ラテン語と英語の違いは，たとえば，Terminologia Anatomica や os longum のように形容詞が名詞に後置することである．これから「医学英語の常識」も読んで，楽しみながら日常英語とは異なる医学英語の特徴を学び，習得に役立ててほしい[1]．

3. 医学英語の構造について
　ほとんどの医学英語は，接頭辞＋語根（→連結形）＋接尾辞で構成されている．刻々と新発見があり，著しく発展を続ける医学においては，用語も増

The Skeletal System

加の一途をたどり，膨大な医学英語が必要とされる．その際，各構成要素の切り貼り自由自在なギリシア語・ラテン語から造語するのが便宜である[2]．また科学の1分野である医学では簡潔な表現が望ましいし，特に医療の場は病気と闘う戦場のようなものである．たとえば骨膜炎を説明的に the inflammation of the membrane around the bones（骨周辺の膜の炎症）というのと，一言で periostinum というのとどちらがよいだろう．periostinum だ！　といった人は，もう医学英語にハマってますよ．

注

1) 英語としての発音に注意．TA がラテン語であるためにたとえば，aorta（大動脈）を【アオータ】，dementia（認知症）を【デメンチア】のように発音する場合があるが，英語ではそれぞれ［eɪɔ́ːtə］［dɪménʃ(i)ə］と発音する．
2) 医学英語の構成要素については後述（p.30）．巻末 Appendix 参照．

医学英語のルーツ―ギリシア神話（1）
atlas（環椎）は Atlas（アトラース）から

2本足で歩く人体には，大きな脳を収めた頭の重さを曲線を描く脊柱が吸収するという特徴がある．その脊柱が頭蓋の後頭骨に入り込んだ部分を環椎（the atlas），第二頸椎を軸椎（the axis）とよぶ．環椎は不動であるのに頭が上下左右に動くのは，この軸椎の上部にある歯突起が環椎に入り込んでいるからだ．

さて，かつて地図帳（atlas）の見返し部分に，ひとりの男が肩に天球を背負った姿があったものだ．この怪力男の名はアトラース（Atlas）．ギリシア神話に登場する巨神族ティターン（Titan）のひとりである．ではなぜ，環椎と同じ名称なのだろう？

それは，まだ神々が権力闘争に明け暮れていた時代にさかのぼる．ギリシア神話によると，世界のはじまりは光も形も何もなく，無限で空漠としたカオス（chaos）が拡がっていたとされる．まず広大な大地の女神ガイア（Gaia）が生まれ，同時に地の奥深く朦朧とした冥界タルタロス，美しい性愛エロスが生まれた[1]．

やがてガイアはエロスに恋し，天空の神ウラノス（Uranos）を産む．ウラノスは母であり妻であるガイアと交わり巨神族のティターンが誕生していく．「それでは近親相姦ではないですか!!」と非難しないで．ここには，この世の生きとし生けるものすべて母なる大地から生じた，という考え方が世界中の神話によく見られるのだから．

しかしウラノスは，子供たちが生まれると悉く，世界の奥深く深く霧が渦巻く冥界に追いやったのだ．夫の（息子の？）あまりの横暴に憤り，ガイアは子供たちに金剛石の斧で「お父さんを殺っておしまい」と唆す．子供たちは皆怖がって引いてしまったが，末子のクロノス（Cronos）は豪胆であった．ある日，星々が光を放つ黒いマントをまとった父がいつものようにふらっとやってきてガイアを覆い，ことを終えるとグハグハと眠ってしまった，その時を狙ってそっと近づき，斧を彼の生殖器めがけて思い切り打ち下ろした！天空の神の生殖器だから，きっととてつもなく大きかったに違いない．海に沈んで無数の白い泡（精子？）が海面に上り，ざわざわと波となって海辺に

The Skeletal System

打ち寄せた．その泡から，あの美の女神アフロディテが誕生したという．

　クロノスは父を幽冥に追放し，第二代権力者になった．彼は世界に秩序をもたらす時の神，農耕の神だから世界はこれで落ち着いた，と思いきや，妻レアとの間に生まれた子供を即座に飲み込んでしまう[2]．「お前も子供にヤラレルだろう」という父の最期の言葉が強迫観念のように刷りこまれてしまったのだ．レアは一計を案じ，第六子のゼウスが生まれると，石をむつきに包んで夫に手渡した．彼はいつものように大急ぎでそれを呑み込み，一安心．一方，ゼウスはエーゲ海のクレタ島で密かに育てられ，勇猛果敢な青年に成長し，父と対決する．彼は父の腹を思いっきり蹴りあげ，出てきた兄弟姉妹たちと力を合わせて勝利を収めると，ギリシア最大のオリュンポスの神々の最高神として世界に君臨するのである．

　この時，クロノス側についたのがアトラース．しかも向う見ずな戦い振りが目立ち，ゼウスの怒りは収まらず「世界の西の果てで天空の端っこを背負っておれ！」と刑が言い渡されたということである．

　このアトラスに因んで第一頸椎である環椎も頭の重さに耐えている故，the atlas と命名されたのである．神話なんぞ非科学的で医学には関係ない！と考える科学的頭脳の持ち主である皆さん，この環椎をそう名付けた解剖学者は，想像力豊かで，しかも知的だとは思いませんか？

注
1) 同時に，幽冥界エレボスと漆黒の夜の女神ニュクス（Nyx）から，矛盾するようだが光り輝くアイテールと昼の女神ヘーメラが生まれ，次にニュクスは健気にもひとりで闘争，運命，死，睡眠，夢，報い，悲運，苦痛，老いという9つの神格を存在させる．生殖に男が不要だったとは，まるで現代医学を地でいくようなもの．
2) 原始社会の食人行為が反映されているともいう．

| Atlas, Cronos, Aphrodite などに因む医学英語 |

　　atlantodidymus　二頭奇形（ひとつの頸と身体にふたつの頭がある双生児）
　　atlantoaxial joint　環軸関節

atlantodontoid　環椎歯突起の

chronic　慢性（ギリシア語の khronos は"時間"の意味）　cf. acute 急性，subacute　亜急性

chronic fatigue syndrome（CFS）　慢性疲労症候群（脱力感，疲労感が6ヶ月以上続く原因不明の症候群）

ether　エーテル（ギリシア神話で天地創造の初期に生じた神格．Aithēr（アイテール））

noctouria　夜尿症（Chaos の娘，夜の女神．Nyx はローマ神話で Nox）

nyctophobia　暗所恐怖症（-phobia：phobos は恐怖症．～嫌い）
　反意語～ philia ＝～の傾向，病的愛向

titanium　チタン（ティターン（Titarn）はウラノスとガイアの間に生まれた巨神たち）

uranoschisis　口蓋裂

hermaphrodite　半陰陽（アフロディテとヘルメスの子供で，入浴中にニンフ（nymph）のひとりと一体となって両性具有となった，と伝えられる）

aphrodisiac　性欲亢進．特に過度の場合．aphro- は泡の意味

CHAPTER 3
The Muscular System　筋肉系

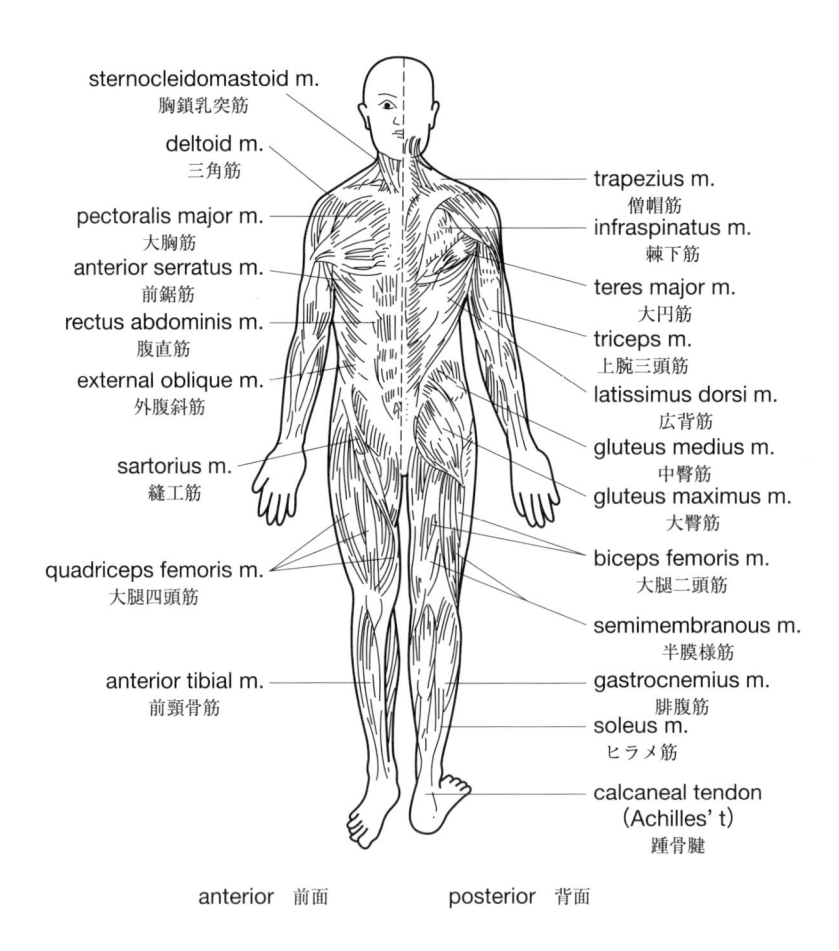

sternocleidomastoid m.
胸鎖乳突筋

deltoid m.
三角筋

pectoralis major m.
大胸筋

anterior serratus m.
前鋸筋

rectus abdominis m.
腹直筋

external oblique m.
外腹斜筋

sartorius m.
縫工筋

quadriceps femoris m.
大腿四頭筋

anterior tibial m.
前頸骨筋

trapezius m.
僧帽筋

infraspinatus m.
棘下筋

teres major m.
大円筋

triceps m.
上腕三頭筋

latissimus dorsi m.
広背筋

gluteus medius m.
中臀筋

gluteus maximus m.
大臀筋

biceps femoris m.
大腿二頭筋

semimembranous m.
半膜様筋

gastrocnemius m.
腓腹筋

soleus m.
ヒラメ筋

calcaneal tendon
(Achilles' t)
踵骨腱

anterior　前面　　posterior　背面

24

Tendon

Background Information

Muscles make up almost 50% of our body weight. When muscles work they contract — become shorter and thicker. When muscles attached to bones contract, they exert a pull on the bones and cause them to move. Most muscles work in pairs — one set works while the other set rests.

綴りに注意

Voluntary muscles move and work when we want them to do so. The muscles of the arm, muscles of the leg, and the neck muscles are examples of voluntary muscles. This kind of muscles has cells that are long, round, and cross-striped (striated).

随意筋

横紋の

Involuntary muscles keep on doing their work whether we think about them or not. The nervous system controls involuntary muscles almost exclusively. The work of the stomach, intestines, lungs, and other internal organs is done by involuntary muscles. This kind of muscles has cells that are slender, smooth, and without cross-stripes. Involuntary muscles are often called smooth muscles.

不随意筋

平滑筋

A third kind of muscle is the cardiac muscle. Cells of the heart are striated both crossways and longways. Tendons attach muscles to bones. This connective tissue is very strong and flexible.

〔出典 A, p.ii : R5 〜 R27〕

Tendon — 腱

Tendon, also called *sinew*, is a strong white cord that attaches muscles to bones. Muscles move bones by pulling on tendons. A tendon is a bundle of many tough fibers. Some tendons are round, others long or flat. One end of a tendon arises from the end of

束
強い繊維
起始する

25

The Muscular System

Biceps muscle of arm　上腕二頭筋

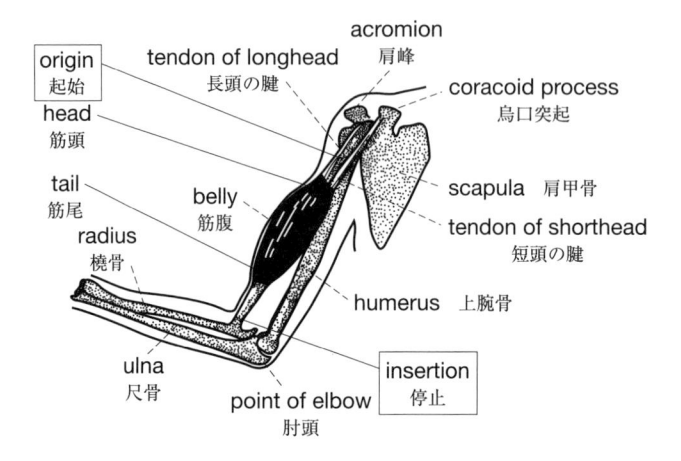

```
origin          tendon of longhead    acromion
起始             長頭の腱              肩峰
head                                          coracoid process
筋頭                                           烏口突起
tail             belly                 scapula  肩甲骨
筋尾             筋腹                  tendon of shorthead
radius                                         短頭の腱
橈骨
                                       humerus  上腕骨
        ulna                insertion
        尺骨                 停止
              point of elbow
              肘頭
```

a muscle.　The other end is woven into the substance　　組み入る
of a bone.　The tendon may slide up and down inside
a sheath of fibrous tissue, as an arm moves in a coat　　繊維組織
sleeve.　A cut tendon can be *sutured* (sewed) together.　　縫合される
Healing may take six weeks or more.

Ligament — 靭帯

　　Ligament is fibrous tissue that holds organs of the
body in place and fastens bones together.　Ligaments
are grouped together in cords, bands, or sheets.
They are as strong as rope.　A *sprain* occurs when lig-　　捻挫
aments covering a joint are torn or twisted.　A
sprained ankle is the partial tearing of the ligaments
that bind the bones of the lower leg to the bones of　　下肢
the foot.　Ligaments heal slowly.　They may never
heal if they are completely torn apart.　Treatment of
sprained ligaments may include exercise, supportive

26

bandages or splints, or even surgery, depending on the ligaments involved and the severity of the injury.

副木（ふくぼく）
〔出典 B, Vol. 12, p.281：R8〜R19〕

Movement — 運動

Movement consists sometimes of locomotion, sometimes of movements of parts of the body, sometimes of changes in the size of openings, and sometimes of propulsion of substances through tubes, for example. Propulsion of blood through arteries by heart movements is one example of the latter. Passage of food through the digestive tract by contractions of the stomach and intestines is another. By means of locomotion, adjustments are made to the external environment. Desirable objects are approached, and undesirable or dangerous ones are repelled. By means of internal movements, vital adjustments and processes are accomplished. Consider the following examples: contraction and relaxation of the iris muscles which allow just the right amount of light to enter the eyes, contractions of the digestive tract muscles which promote digestion and elimination, and contractions of the heart which keep the blood circulating.

歩行運動

推進力

消化管

追い払われる・拒否される
生命維持に必要な

虹彩

促進する

注）muscle は（14 世紀に名づけられた）ラテン語の musculus（ハツカネズミ）に由来し，cle（＝小さい，細いを表す接尾辞）が付加された．筋肉の動くさまがネズミに似ていることから．

The Muscular System

Kinds of movements 運動

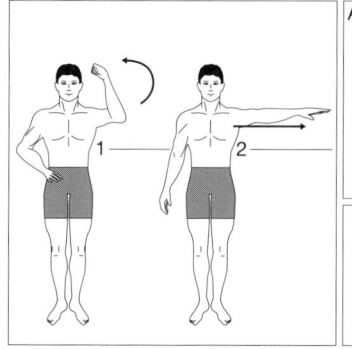

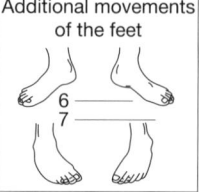

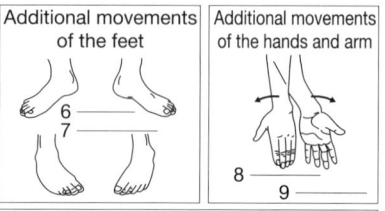

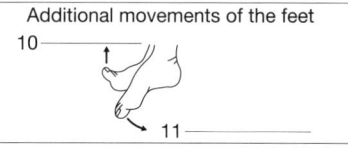

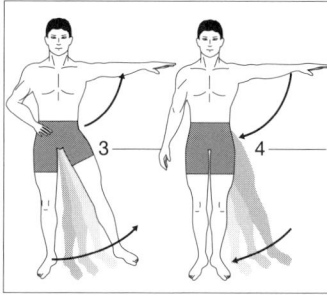

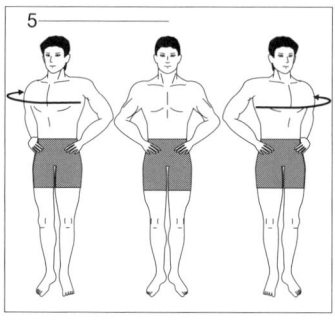

1. flexion 屈曲
2. extension 伸展
3. abduction 外転
4. adduction 内転
5. rotation 回転
6. eversion 外返し
7. inversion 内返し
8. pronation 回内
9. supination 回外
10. dorsiflexion 背屈
11. plantar flexion 底屈

Movement

Let's pronounce medical English terms.

1. triceps muscle
2. muscle fiber
3. striated muscle
4. sprain

Review questions

1. Of what substance are tendon and ligament made up?
2. If ligament is damaged, what will happen?
3. Write the name of muscle below in Japanese and select the appropriate explanation for each tissue.

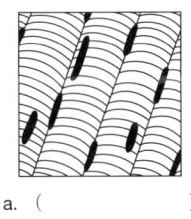

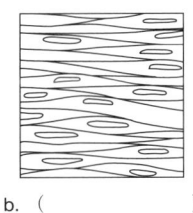

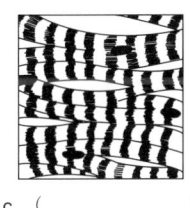

a. (　　　　　)　　b. (　　　　　)　　c. (　　　　　)

1) This kind of muscles has cells that are long, round, and cross-striped.
2) This kind of muscles has cells that are slender, smooth, and without cross-stripes.
3) This kind of muscles has cells of the heart are striated both crossways and longways.

The Muscular System

医学英語の常識（3）
医学英語の構成

現在の辞書に掲載されている英単語のうち，本来の英語は 25％程度，50％はラテン語系，10％がギリシア語系である．医学英語に関してはほとんどがギリシア語，ラテン語から借入したものである．そのため，膨大な医学英語の習得には，その用語特有の構成パターンを覚えることが医学英語習得の早道であるといえる．なお，頻用される各要素例を Appendix に掲載した．

医学英語の多くは，「接頭辞＋連結形（語根）＋接尾辞」で構成される．それぞれの要素の役割は，

1. 接頭辞（prefix，略語 pref.）
   語のはじめにおかれ，後続の語の意味を変える．
   例：abnormal（異常な）→接頭辞 ab- ＋連結系 norm ＋接尾辞 -al
2. 連結形（combining form，略語 comb. form）
   一語＋母音（combining vowel）
   ただし，母音ではじまる語の前は連結母音の o は省かれる．接辞とは別に独立性をもち，しかも他の語と結合する．
   例：gastrectomy（胃切除）→連結形 gastr-（胃）＋連結系 ectom（切除）＋接尾辞 -y
3. 語根（word root）
   語の基底（base）となるもので，すべての語は語根をもっている．
   例：leukocyte（白血球）→連結形 leuko-（白い）＋語根 cyte（細胞）
4. 接尾辞（suffix，略語 suf.）
   前の語の品詞を変える．
   例：respiration（呼吸）→接頭辞 re-（反復）＋連結形 spiro-（呼吸）＋接尾辞 -tion

原則として，接頭辞，接尾辞はギリシア語にはギリシア語根の，ラテン語にはラテン語根に結合し造語される．

さて，練習問題として，世界で一番長い単語である
　　　　　　　pneumonoultramicroscopicsilicovolcanoconiosis
を構成要素に分析してみよう．

　pneumono-（連結形）肺
　ultra-（接頭辞）極端な，過度の
　micro-（連結形）小・微
　-scop（連結形）鏡
　-ic（接尾辞）見る・観察する，〜に関する
　silico-（連結形）ケイ素の
　volcano-（連結形）激しい
　coni（語根）塵埃
　-osis（接尾辞）病的状態

　まとめると，「肺に過度に（顕微鏡で観察されうるほど）微細なケイ素の塵埃が爆発的に（貯留する）病的状態」となる．病名は「じん肺症」（実際には，pneumoconiosis, coniosis と省略するので安心してほしい）．
　医学英語なんて恐くない，である

The Muscular System

医学英語のルーツ―ギリシア神話（2）
踵(かかと)の腱は，ギリシア神話の英雄アキレウスのアキレス腱

　英語の背景にある西欧文明の支柱はヘブライ文化とギリシア文化であるといわれ，そしてその遺産は前者が聖書，後者がギリシア神話であることはいうまでもないだろう．両書に語られた物語や言葉は，かの文豪 W. シェイクスピアの劇中のセリフと同様に西欧の人々の生活に浸透し，その精神的な糧となってきた．

　さて，踵にある丈夫な腱，踵骨腱（calcaneal tendon）を別称アキレス腱[1]（Achilles tendon）という．その語源となった Achilles [əkíli:z] もまたこのギリシア神話に登場する勇将であるが，川の女神テティスと人間ペレウスとの間に生まれた半神半人であった．

　当時ギリシア世界では，子が生まれる時に神の託宣を伺うのが習わしであったが，アキレウスは「戦いに出れば必ず死ぬ」という託宣を受けた．

　母テティスは神託を避けようと，アキレウスの足首をもってステュクス川[2]に何度も浸した[3]．赤ん坊の泣き声に気づいたペレウスが思わず「何をしている！」と叫んだものだから，妻は驚いて川へ逃げ帰ってしまった．父親も又，我が子を死から守るためにエーゲ海の島で女の子として養育係に育てさせた．しかし，物売りが店開きをした時に，彼が刀を手にとったので男であるとばれてしまう．勇壮果敢な父と，女神である母の遺伝子だけでも十分強い．さらに養育係は肝臓やモツ等をよく食べさせた．というわけで，武術に秀でた若者に成長した．そして，実際にギリシアとトロイアとの戦い[4]に親友の敵(かたき)を取ろうと出陣し，神託の通りに戦死したのである．

　10年にも及んだトロイ戦争だが，そもそものきっかけはアキレウスの両親の結婚式だった．神々，人間が一堂に会した盛大な結婚式に招待されない女神がいた．ゼウスと妻ヘラの娘で争いの女神エリスである．確かに彼女は不和や争いを起こしては，しかもそれに快感を覚えるという困った性格であった．案の定，結婚式に招待されずムカッときた彼女は，ここでも争いの種を播いた．醜男(ぶおとこ)で名工，あの美と豊穣の女神アフロディテの夫ヘパイストスの造った黄金の林檎を盗み，「世界で一番美しい女に」と書いて祝宴に投げ込んで．

花嫁を差し置いて，一番はわたし，と主張した三人の女神がいた．ゼウスの妻，縁結びの女神ヘラ，兜をかぶり，盾を持ってゼウスの頭から生まれた知恵と戦いの女神アテナ，そしてアフロディテであった．ゼウスは審判をと攻め寄られたが，賢い．後の災いを恐れて，牧神パリスに委ねて逃げた．すると女神たちは，パリスを賄賂で買収しにかかった．ヘラはアジアの王を，アテナは戦争の勝利と知恵を，アフロディテは人間の女の中で最も美しいと評判のヘレネーを約束したのだが，さて，これを読んでいる男性の方々は，どれを望むだろうか？ パリスはヘレネーを選んだのだ．これが次の災い．彼女には夫がいたのだから．パリスは夫メネラーオスの留守の間にヘレネーと財宝を奪ってトロイアに戻った[5]．当然，夫はヘレネーを取り戻さなければ立場がない．その結果，戦争が起き，出陣したアキレウスの踵をパリスの矢が射抜き，神託の通りに戦死したのだ．

さて，なぜ足首が？ そう，テティスがステュクス川に浸す時に持った足首だけは不死身にならなかったのだ．それにしても，三人の女神といい，争いの女神エリスといい，人間の絶世の美女ヘレネーといい，女は恐い，ですか？

注
1) アキレウスはギリシア語読み．日本語では通常，アキレスという．
2) 日本でいう三途の川．
3) 一説には，霊験のある仙膏を体に塗って火で焙ったともいわれる．
4) トロイ戦争は，吟遊詩人ホメーロスが語った「イリアド」によって後世の私たちに伝えられた．一言でギリシア神話伝説とよばれる総体を知ることは容易ではない．神話が形態を整えたのは，ローマ帝政時代初期であったらしい．それ以前に，ホメーロスやヘーシオドスの叙事詩によって，オリュンポスの神々を頂点とする体系が形成され，英雄詩が築かれた．
5) 一説にはヘレネーがパリスの美貌に心を奪われたとも．

The Muscular System

Achilles に因む医学英語

Achilles tendon　アキレス腱（図参照）

Achilles bursa　アキレス腱の滑液包

Achillotenotomy　アキレス腱切り（術）

Achilles paratendinitis　アキレス腱周囲炎（アキレス腱には滑膜性腱鞘はないが，代わりに周囲を覆う結合組織パラテノンがある）

Achilles（tendon）reflex　アキレス腱反射（アキレス腱をハンマーで叩いたとき，腓腹筋に生じる収縮）

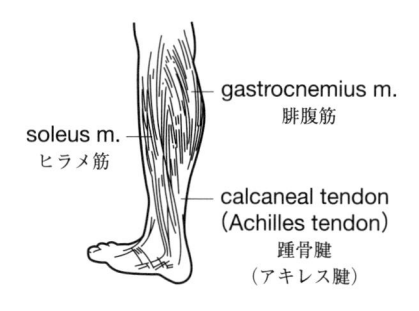

gastrocnemius m.
腓腹筋

soleus m.
ヒラメ筋

calcaneal tendon
(Achilles tendon)
踵骨腱
（アキレス腱）

CHAPTER 4
The Circulatory System　循環系

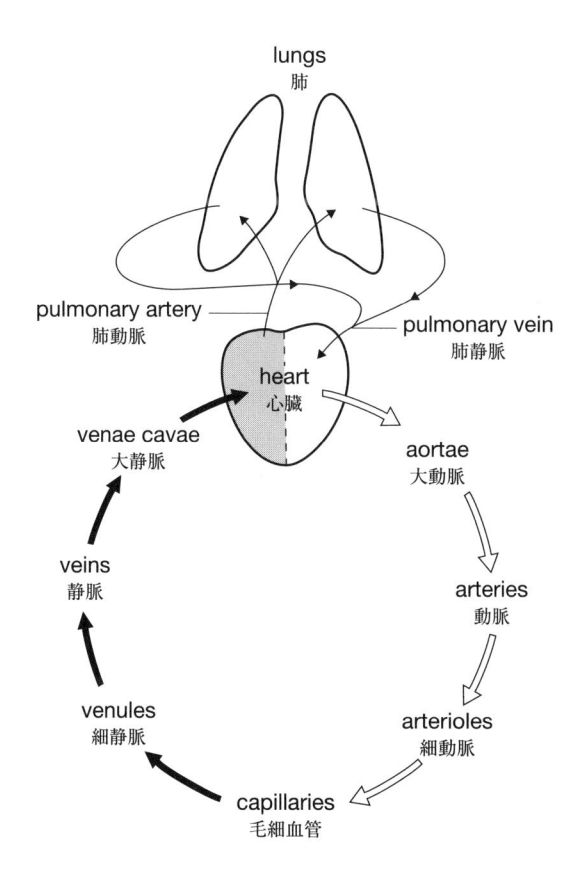

```
                    lungs
                     肺

pulmonary artery              pulmonary vein
    肺動脈                          肺静脈
                    heart
 venae cavae        心臓
    大静脈
                                  aortae
                                  大動脈

  veins
   静脈
                                 arteries
                                  動脈

  venules
  細静脈
                                arterioles
                                  細動脈
              capillaries
               毛細血管
```

注）肺動脈, 肺静脈の血管名に注意. O_2, CO_2 含有に関係なく, 心臓を基準にして, 心臓からでる血管はすべて動脈, 入る血管は静脈である.

The Circulatory System

Background Information

The circulatory system consists of the heart, the blood vessels, and blood. The heart is a muscular organ that rhythmically contracts, forcing the blood through a system of vessels. Those vessels that carry blood away from the heart are known as arteries.

血管 (vessel=tube)

Vessels that carry blood to the heart are known as veins. The larger veins below the levels of the heart have to prevent the backward flow of the blood. The small vessels that make up the network of channels between the arteries and veins are known as capillaries. When the left ventricle of the heart contracts, the blood is forced to flow out and into the body's largest artery, the aorta. Branches from the aorta carry the blood upward to the head and downward to the body's trunk and extremities.

〔véin〕

〔eiɔ́ːtə〕

体幹と四肢

An area of an artery dilates when surge of blood enters and then contracts forcing the blood forward. Dissolved oxygen from the lungs and food materials are carried by the blood to the cells via the capillaries. Wastes are picked up from the cells. The capillaries unite to form larger vessels, veins, which carry the blood to the heart.

老廃物

The blood is the fluid portion of the circulatory system. Blood consists of a solid part, the cells, and the liquid part, the plasma. The red blood cells carry oxygen from the lungs and carbon dioxide to the lungs. White blood cells destroy bacteria and help repair tissues. The plasma consists of proteins and dissolved salts in water.

血漿

タンパク質〔próutiːn〕

〔出典 A, p.iv : R1 〜 R27〕

The constitution of the blood　血液の成分

1. cells 血球（formed elements 有形成分）
    a. red blood cells, or erythrocytes 赤血球　5,000,000/mm^3
    b. white blood cells, or leukocytes 白血球　7,000-9,000/mm^3
      （1）granular leukocytes 顆粒球
        (a) neutrophils 好中球（53.5%）
        (b) eosinophils 好酸球（3%）
        (c) basophils 好塩基球（0.5%）
      （2）nongranular leukocytes 非顆粒球
        (a) lymphocytes リンパ球（38%）
        (b) monocytes 単球（5%）
    c. platelets 血小板　200,000-800,000/mm^3
2. plasma 血漿（liquid element 液体成分）

注
1) /mm^3 は per one cubic millimeter と読む．
2) 色彩の英語表現については p.201 参照．
3) 数の接頭辞については p.183 参照．

Let's pronounce medical English terms.

1. aorta　2. vena cava〔víːnə kéivə〕　3. vein　4. capillary
5. erythrocyte　6. corpuscle　7. atrium〔éitriəm〕

Review questions

1. What blood vessel is the thickest?
2. What blood vessel is the smallest?
3. What part of the blood is liquid?
4. What function does the white blood cells perform?
5. Write the medical English which has the same meaning for each word.
    1) red blood cell　（　　　　　　　　）
    2) white blood cell　（　　　　　　　　）
6. Write the meaning of the underlined part of the following words.
    1) lympho<u>cyte</u>　　　（　　　　　　）
    2) <u>erythro</u>cyte　　　（　　　　　　）
    3) <u>leuko</u>cyte　　　　（　　　　　　）

The Circulatory System

4) granular leukocyte (   )
5) neutrophil (   )
6) basophil (   )
7) eosinophil (   )
8) monocyte (   )

Heart — 心臓

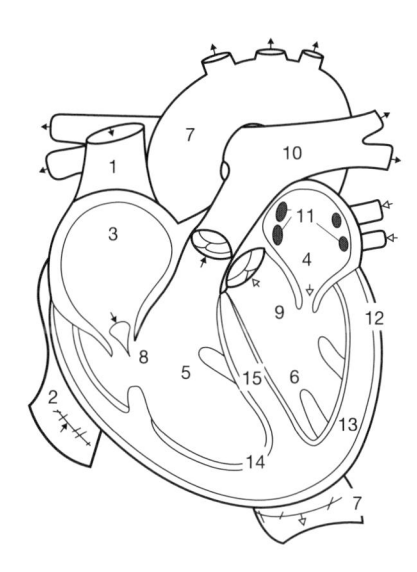

1. superior vena cava　上大静脈
2. inferior vena cava　下大静脈
3. right atrium　右心房
4. left atrium　左心房
5. right ventricle　右心室
6. left ventricle　左心室
7. aorta　大動脈
8. tricuspid valve　三尖弁
9. mitral valve（bicuspid valve）　僧帽弁（二尖弁）
10. pulmonary artery　肺動脈
11. pulmonary vein　肺静脈
12. epicardium　心外膜
13. myocardium　心筋層
14. endocardium　心内膜
15. septum　中隔

注）英単語が骨格や部位，位置の英語から構成されていることに注目する．

The Circulatory System

Background Information

If you cut open a heart you can see many of its main structural features. It is hollow, not solid. A partition (the septum) divides it into right and left sides. It has four cavities inside: a small upper cavity (*atrium*) and a larger lower cavity (ventricle) on each side. Cardiac muscle tissue composes the wall of the heart; it is usually referred to as the *myocardium*. Myocarditis, therefore, means inflammation of the heart muscle. A very smooth tissue, endocardium, lines the cavity of the heart. Endocarditis, of course, means inflammation of the heart lining. This condition can cause rough spots to develop in the endocardium, which may lead to thrombosis.

 The heart has a covering as well as a lining. Its covering, the pericardium, consists of two layers of fibrous tissue with a small space in between. The inner layer of the pericardium covers the heart like an apple skin covers an apple, but the outer layer fits around the heart like a loose fitting sack, allowing enough room for the heart to beat in it. These two pericardial layers slip against each other without friction when the heart beats because they are moist, not dry surfaces. ... A thin film of pericardial fluid furnishes the lubricating moistness between the heart and its enveloping pericardial sac.

 The heart expands and contracts by the force of the muscle (the myocardium) under impulse from the sinoatrial node, and a normal heart beats about 70 times a minute; the contracting beat as it pumps blood out (the systole) is followed by a weaker diasto-

---

空洞の
中隔

心房，心室

心筋組織
心筋とよばれる

心内膜炎

ざらざらした発疹
血栓症

被覆
心膜，線維組織

ゆったりした袋

摩擦

心膜液
滑らかにする湿気

同房結節（心拍を制約するペースメーカー）
心収縮期　〔sístəli〕
心拡張期　〔daiǽstəli〕

le, where the muscles relax to allow blood to flow back into the heart.

In a heart attack, part of the myocardium is deprived of blood because of a clot in a coronary artery; this has an effect on the rhythm of the heartbeat and can be fatal. In heart block, impulses from the sino-atrial node fail to reach the ventricles properly; there are either longer impulses (first degree block) or missing impulses (second degree block) or no impulses at all (complete heart block), in which case the ventricles continue to beat slowly and independently of the S-A node.

Let's pronounce medical English terms.

1. vena cava 2. atrium 3. pulmonary vein
4. aorta 5. systole (発音注意) 6. sinoarterilal

Review questions

1. Give the names of four cavities inside the heart.
2. How many valves are there inside the heart?
3. Why does the heart have no friction when it beats?
4. Translate the sentences below into Japanese.
   Your heart. ...
   1) is a busy pump linked by 160,000 kilometers of pipelines to all parts of your body.
   2) weights less than 0.5 kilograms.
   3) is as big as your fist.
   4) beats about 70 times a minute, and more than 100,000 times in a single day.
   5) pumps 4.7 liters of blood through its chambers every 60 seconds.

The Circulatory System

    6) does enough work in one hour to lift a weight of 1.4 metric tons more than 30 centimeters off the ground.

5. Write English terms that matches Japanese on the right.
   1) (　　　　　) vena cava　　上大静脈
   2) right (　　　　　)　　　　右心房
   3) (　　　　　) valve　　　　肺動脈弁
   4) pulmonary (　　　　　)　　肺動脈
   5) (　　　　　) valve　　　　大動脈弁

6. Write the meaning of the underlined part of each word in Japanese, but if possible in English.
   1) <u>cardi</u>ac muscle　(　　　　　)
   2) <u>myo</u>cardium　　 (　　　　　)
   3) myocard<u>itis</u>　　 (　　　　　)
   4) end<u>o</u>cardium　　 (　　　　　)
   5) <u>peri</u>cardial sac　(　　　　　)

医学英語の常識(4)
複数形

　医学英語の複数形には，ギリシア語，ラテン語からの借入語の場合，規則性がある．その一般的法則には，以下のような代表的な形がある．

1. um で終わる単語は a に変える．
   bacterium → bacteria（細菌）
   cranium → crania（頭蓋骨）
   ovum → ova（卵子）
2. a で終わる単語は a に e をつける．
   ulna → ulnae（尺骨）
   scapula → scapulae（肩甲骨）
   vertebra → vertebrae（椎骨）
3. us で終わる単語は us を i に変える．
   bacillus → bacilli（桿菌）
   nervus → nervi（神経）
   villus → villi（絨毛）　例外：sinus → sinus（洞）
4. is で終わる単語は is を es に変える．
   dialysis → dialyses（透析）
   peristalsis → peristalses（蠕動）
   pericardiocentesis → pericardiocenteses（心膜穿刺）
   変形：iris → irides（虹彩）
5. ix, ex で終わる単語は ix, ex を ices に変える．
   appendix → appendices（appendixes）（虫垂）
   cortex → cortices（皮質）
   helix → helices（耳輪）
6. on で終わる単語は on を a に変える．
   ganglion → ganglia（神経節）
   myelencephalon → myelencephala（または〜s）（髄脳）
   spermatozoon → spermatozoa（精子）

The Circulatory System

医学英語のルーツ―ギリシア神話（3）
その一言が…？　英雄ペルセウスと「メドゥーサの頭」（Medusa head）

　肝臓は身体にとって「肝心肝要」だし，liverがあるから生きている（live）．この肝臓が肝硬変（cirrhosis）になると，「メドゥーサの頭」とよばれる病態を引き起こす場合がかつてみられた．

　メドゥーサは清らかな美しい娘たち，ゴルゴン三姉妹のひとりであったが，メドゥーサが光の輪が輝く毛髪をつい自慢してしまったのだ．それを耳にした女神アテナの逆鱗に触れてしまった．冷酷にもメドゥーサの自慢の髪を蛇に変えてしまった．それでも気がすまず，この世のものとは思えない醜い顔に変え，それでも気が収まらず，目を見たものは誰でも石になってしまうようにしたのだ．

　さて，「このメドゥーサの頭をとってくる」と断言したのは勇猛果敢な若者ペルセウスである．なぜ，そういうことになったのか？

　ペルセウスの母はダナエである．彼女は楚々として美しい娘に成長し，恋をした．恋すると脳下垂体からホルモンが分泌され，目や皮膚の粘膜は潤い，美しく輝く．ところがダナエが産む男子に殺されるという神託を受けていた彼女の父は，苦慮したあげく，娘を青銅の塔に幽閉して男を近づけないようにした．高い窓から見えるのは空と雲ばかり．吹きわたる風と語らいながら時を過ごす彼女のことが，女好きのゼウス神の耳に達した．彼は変幻自在な神．黄金の雨となって塔の窓からダナエに降り注ぎ，彼女はとうとうペルセウスを懐妊した．父王は驚愕したが，天使のような赤ん坊を殺すに忍びなく，小さな空気穴をあけた箱に二人を入れ，小船にのせて地中海に流したのである．

　母の心は強靭であった．我が子をしっかりと胸に抱き，流れに身を任せているうちに運よくセリポス島に漂着した．島の王の弟は温厚な性質で二人を暖かく守ったのだが，兄王は，わがまま，強欲な性分であった．逆境に耐えて深い憂いを湛え，百合のように香気を放ち，しかも子を産んだばかりの母性の美しさをにじませるダナエにぞっこん惚れ込んでしまった．でも，貞淑で誇り高い彼女は勿論ステータスに心を売るなんてことはしない．

　島の秋祭りの日，集まり祝う人々は王に貢物をささげた．貧しいペルセウス母子には贈り物がない．母親思いの彼は思わず「メドゥーサの頭を取って

医学英語のルーツ—ギリシア神話 (3)

差し上げましょう」と断言してしまったのだ．その一言が身の破滅……となるだろうとばかり，王は内心大喜び．

さて，母思いの彼に，体が見えなくなる羊の皮衣，メドゥーサの顔を見なくてすむ盾と，首を刎ねる剣を手渡したのは女神アテナ．女の美には過剰反応するアテナなのに勇気ある美少年には肩入れする？ いえ，彼の成長を見守る優しく賢明な女神でもあった．さらに男神ヘルメスが飛ぶように走る靴を貸してくれたので，ペルセウスは，ゴルゴン三姉妹が住む地の果てに瞬く間にたどり着き，くねくね身を捩り，赤い舌をチロチロ，シューシューと音をさせるメドゥーサの蛇の髪と恐ろしい顔を見ないように盾で顔を隠し，頭をぶっ千切ったのであった．

このあとのいくつかの冒険談は省略．途中，彼はアフリカでアンドロメダを苦境から救い出して妻とし，母のもとに戻った．王に約束通りにメドゥーサの顔を差し出すと，当然，王も石となってしまった．彼は母と妻と三人で祖父の国へと旅立つ．めでたし，めでたし……のはずだが，神託は必ず実現する．旅の途中，ある地で競技大会に参加し，投げた円盤が偶々見物をしていた祖父アクリシオスに命中してしまった．

このように，長いメドゥーサの頭をめぐる話は，ペルセウスのその一言が身の破滅，とはならなかったものの，祖父は神託を逃れられなかった，と神話は伝える．

注）因みに Caput Medusae の病態は，"The Caput Medusae is found more often in textbook than in cirrhosis of the liver."（「メドゥーサの頭」は肝硬変よりも多く教科書に見られる）である．

Caput Medusae に因む医学英語

Caput Medusae（Medusa head） メドゥーサの頭：瘢痕，繊維症が門脈圧を高める結果，門脈亢進が生じ，大量の血液は胎児循環の名残である肝円索から臍傍静脈へ流れる．重症の場合，浅腹壁静脈が臍周辺の静脈と合流し，皮膚下で膨れ上がる．まるで細い蛇が四方に広がっているように見え，ギリシア神話に登場する蛇の毛髪をもつメドゥーサを想起させること

The Circulatory System

から，「メドゥーサの頭」（Medusa head あるいは Caput Medusae）とよばれる．
occipital　後頭の
biceps　二頭筋
capillary　毛細血管（caput 頭 + pilus 毛）
capsule　被膜
caput femoris　大腿骨頭
caput long　長骨頭

CHAPTER 5
The Lymphatic System　リンパ系

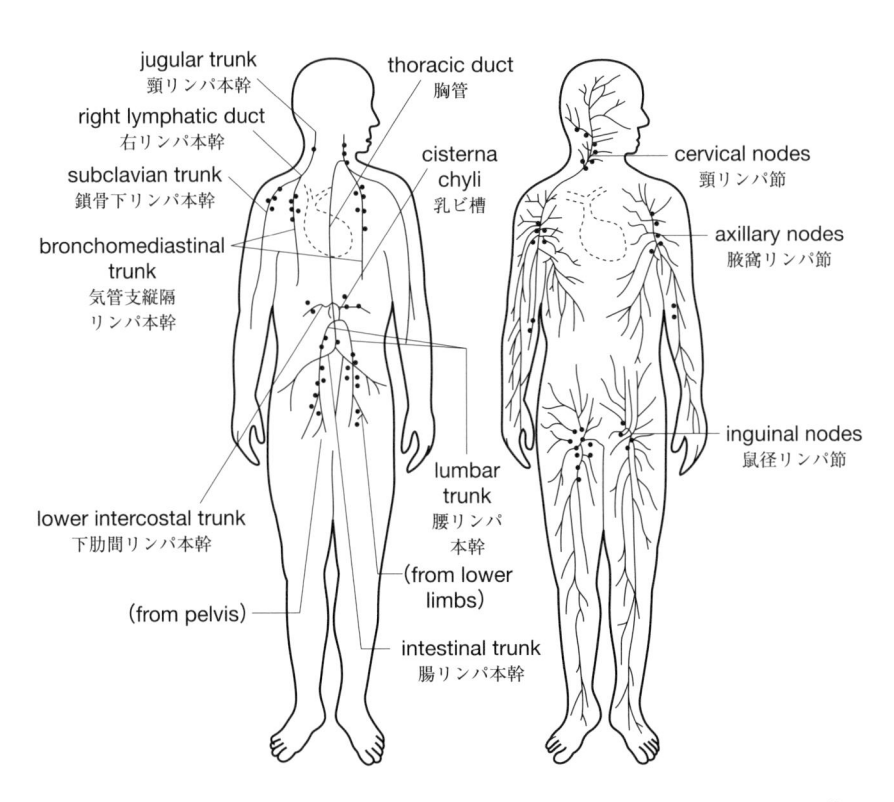

Deep lymph nodes
深在性リンパ節

Superficial lymph nodes
浅在性リンパ節

jugular trunk
頸リンパ本幹

thoracic duct
胸管

right lymphatic duct
右リンパ本幹

cisterna chyli
乳ビ槽

subclavian trunk
鎖骨下リンパ本幹

cervical nodes
頸リンパ節

bronchomediastinal trunk
気管支縦隔
リンパ本幹

axillary nodes
腋窩リンパ節

inguinal nodes
鼠径リンパ節

lumbar trunk
腰リンパ本幹

lower intercostal trunk
下肋間リンパ本幹

(from lower limbs)

(from pelvis)

intestinal trunk
腸リンパ本幹

The Lymphatic System

Background Information

Lymphatic system is a network of small vessels that resemble blood vessels. The lymphatic system returns fluid from body tissues to the blood stream. This process is necessary because fluid pressure in the body continuously causes water, proteins, and other materials to seep out of tiny blood vessels called *capillaries*. The fluid that has leaked out, called *interstitial fluid*, bathes and nourishes body tissues.

If there were no way for excess interstitial fluid to return to the blood, the tissues would become swollen. Most of the extra fluid seeps into capillaries that have low fluid pressure. The rest returns by way of the lymphatic system and is called *lymph*. Some scientists consider the lymphatic system to be part of the circulatory system because lymph comes from the blood and returns to the blood.

The lymphatic system also serves as one of the body's defenses against infection. Harmful particles and bacteria that have entered the body are filtered out by small masses of tissue along the lymphatic vessels. These bean-shaped accumulations are called *lymph nodes*.

網目構造

血流

タンパク質
血管
漏れ出る, 間質液

膨張する
しみ入る

リンパ液

感染防御
細菌

リンパ節

Structure of the lymph node ― リンパ節の構造

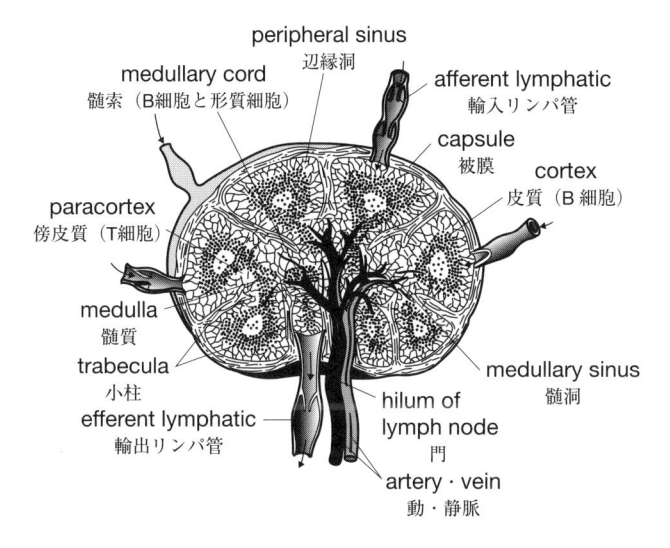

```
                    peripheral sinus
                        辺縁洞
     medullary cord            afferent lymphatic
     髄索（B細胞と形質細胞）        輸入リンパ管
                              capsule
                               被膜
                                     cortex
                                     皮質（B細胞）
     paracortex
     傍皮質（T細胞）

     medulla
     髄質
     trabecula
     小柱                      medullary sinus
                              髄洞
     efferent lymphatic
     輸出リンパ管      hilum of
                    lymph node
                      門
                   artery・vein
                    動・静脈
```

Parts of the lymphatic system ― リンパ系の部位

 Lymphatic vessels, like blood vessels, are found throughout the body. Lymph flows from tiny vessels with many branches into larger vessels. Eventually, lymph from all but the upper right quarter of the body reaches the *thoracic duct*, the largest lymphatic vessel. The thoracic duct lies along the front of the spine. Lymph flows upward through this duct into a blood vessel near the junction of the neck and the left shoulder. Lymph from the upper right quarter of the body flows into the *right lymphatic ducts* in the right half of the chest. The lymph then drains from these ducts into the bloodstream near the junction of the neck and right shoulder.

 Lymph is chemically much like plasma, the liquid

リンパ管

…以外
胸管

脊柱

右リンパ本幹
流出する

The Lymphatic System

part of the blood. But lymph contains only about half as much protein as plasma, because large protein molecules do not seep through blood vessel walls so easily as do some other substances. Lymph is transparent and straw-colored.

 Lymph nodes may be found at many places along the lymphatic vessels. They look like bumps and have diameters from 1 to 25 millimeters. The term *node* comes from the Latin word *nodus,* meaning *knot,* and lymph nodes resemble knots in a "string" of lymphatic vessels. The nodes are bunched together in certain areas, especially in the neck and armpits, above the groin, and near various organs and large blood vessels. Lymph nodes contain large cells called *macrophages* that absorb harmful matter and dead tissue.

 Lymphocytes are a kind of white blood cell produced in the lymph nodes. They defend the body against infection. When abnormal cells or materials from outside the body pass into the lymph nodes, lymphocytes in the nodes produce substances called *antibodies.* The antibodies either destroy the abnormal or foreign matter or make it harmless. Large numbers of lymphocytes are found in the lymph nodes and in lymph itself. They outnumber all other kinds of cells in lymph.

 Lymphoid tissue resembles the tissue of the lymph nodes. It is found in some parts of the body that are not generally considered part of the lymphatic system. For example, the adenoids and tonsils, the spleen, and the thymus consist of lymphoid tissue. This tis-

透明
淡黄色

こぶ
直径
結節

腋窩
鼠径部

マクロファージ

リンパ球

抗体
異物

…に数で勝る

リンパ様組織

アデノイド，扁桃
胸腺

sue produces and contains lymphocytes, and it aids in the body's defense against infection.

Spleen — 脾臓

The spleen remains one of the mystery organs of the body. Quite a bit of doubt still exists about its functions. The three lower ribs provide a protective shelter over the spleen, which is located in the upper left corner of the abdominal cavity just under the diaphragm. Except for blood vessels and nerves, the spleen connects with no other organs.

保護
腹腔
横隔膜

The spleen's main functions seem to be to form lymphocytes and monocytes (as do the lymph nodes) and to act as the body's blood bank. The spleen can store almost two cups of blood and quickly release it back into circulation when more blood is needed—during strenuous exercise and after hemorrhage, for instance.

激しい運動, 出血

Let's pronounce medical English terms.

1. lymph node   2. lymphatic vessel   3. hemorrhage

Review questions

1. What's the difference between lymphatic vessels and blood vessels?
2. What does the word "node" mean?
3. What substance do lymphocytes produce and what part do they play in the body?
4. What functions does spleen seem to perform?
5. Find the appropriate definition of the words.
   1) lymphocyte   (   )   2) lymph node   (   )
   3) antibody   (   )   4) foreign matter   (   )

The Lymphatic System

5) hemorrhage (   )
   a. an object or piece of extraneous matter that has entered the body by accident or design
   b. a form of leukocyte occurring in the lymphatic tissue which destroys abnormal materials both inside and from outside the body
   c. a severe loss of blood from a ruptured blood tubes inside a person's body
   d. a mass of lymphoid tissue situated in the lymphatic system where lymph is filtered and lymphocytes are produced
   e. a substance that the body produces in the blood to fight disease

Treatment of cancer
癌の治療

Cancer is a life-threatening disease that can strike any person at any age. It can strike with or without warning and has been a recognized disease for more than 100 years. Prevention is the best line of defense. ... If the spread is not controlled or checked, cancer can result in death; however, many cancers can be cured if detected and treated promptly. ... Treatment of cancer is continually changing as new technology develops. ... The physician may recommend one or any combination of treatment procedures to combat a particular form of cancer.

(1) Surgery — 外科手術

Surgery now is more precise because of improved diagnostic equipment and opening procedures and advances in preoperative and postoperative care. 術前,術後のケア
Surgery for cancer may be specific, palliative, or preventive.

Specific surgery is done to remove all of the cancerous tissue and, it is hoped to cure the person. The types of cancers that respond well to this type of surgery are those of the lung, skin, stomach, large intestine, breast, and endometrium. Palliative surgery is 子宮内膜,緩和的外科手術
done to sustain the individual with cancer or to alleviate the pain that directly or indirectly results from the cancer. ... Reconstructive surgery may also be used, especially in the breast, skin, head, and neck cancers. In advanced cancers, palliative surgery may be done to sever nerves to alleviate pain. Preventive surgery 痛みを軽減する

may be done to prevent the development of cancer. For example, polyps of the colon may be removed because they are thought to be precancerous.

ポリープ〔páləp〕

(2) Radiation therapy — 放射線療法

More than half of all persons with cancer receive some type of radiation therapy.　Radiation may be used to cure, to control the disease, or to prevent malignant leukemias from infiltrating the brain or spinal cord.　There are two types of radiation: (1)electromagnetic rays and (2) particles. ...

脊髄

電磁波

The goal of radiation therapy is to destroy as much of the tumor as possible without affecting surrounding healthy tissue. ... The effects of radiation on the body include cell death, because ionizing radiation disrupts DNA and interferes with cell replication and growth.　Recovery from radiation damage to normal tissue does occur between doses, but the degree varies, depending on the radiosensitivity of the normal tissue. ... The adverse effects of radiation generally occur in the skin, mucous membranes, and bone marrow.　Hair may begin to fall out, erythema or redness of the skin may develop, and eating may be difficult because of the nausea, vomiting, and mucosal damage to the mouth and stomach.　These distressing side effects generally subside, either between radiation treatments or after the therapy is complete.

腫瘍

deoxyribonucleic acid：デオキシリボ核酸

骨髄
紅斑

吐き気，嘔吐

(3) Chemotherapy — 化学療法

Chemotherapy may be used alone or in combination with other cancer treatments.　It is especially ef-

(5) Hormonal therapy

fective against cancers that spread, such as leukemias and some solid cancers, including choriocarcinoma ... and Hodgkin's disease.

 The goals of chemotherapy are to cure, to control, or to use as palliative agent. ... Most of these drugs are toxic and have adverse effects on the gastrointestinal tract, skin, and bone marrow. ... The person receiving chemotherapy will be monitored closely with laboratory testing and physical examination to evaluate the efficacy of the treatment and to detect potentially serious side effects.

白血病

絨毛がん（子宮内，まれに睾丸内）

ホジキン病．Thomas Hodgkin（1798-1866）英国人医師

毒性

臨床検査

身体検査

副作用

(4) Immunotherapy（Biotherapy）— 免疫療法（生物学的療法）

 Some tumors overwhelm the body's immune system; radiation and chemotherapy may also suppress the immune system. Thus, treatment to enhance the immune system's response may be indicated. Biotherapy is most effective in the early stages of cancer. The use of interferon, naturally occurring body protein that is capable of killing cancer cells or stopping their growth in high-risk melanomas, has been useful. Bone marrow transplantation has proved effective in restoring hematologic and immunologic properties in clients with some cancers, such as Hodgkin's disease and multiple myeloma. Other transplantations used include peripheral blood stem cell transplantation and cord blood transplantation.

薬物療法

インターフェロン

黒色腫

(5) Hormonal therapy — ホルモン療法

 Hormonal therapy is treatment that adds, blocks, or removes hormones. It is based on research that

55

The Lymphatic System

shows that certain hormone affect the growth of certain cancers. Surgical removal of glands that produce the hormones may be necessary or administration of synthetic hormones may be tried to block the body's natural hormones. ...After breast surgery, drugs such as Tamoxifen or Raloxifene may be prescribed for 5 years. In metastatic prostate cancer, hormonal deprivation therapy is main treatment, especially in men with less advanced prostate cancer. More and more drugs for hormonal therapy are available for physicians to use in the treatment of prostate cancer.

投与，合成ホルモン

タモキシフェン（抗エストロゲン薬の一つ），ラロキシフェン（エストロゲン関連化合物の一つ）
進行性前立腺がん

(6) Alternative therapy ── 代替療法

Increased benefit may be achieved if persons with cancer carefully consider both traditional or conventional treatments and alternative treatment therapies. ...

Alternative practitioners recognize the three major forms of conventional cancer treatment and understand the wisdom of each. Most, however, prefer that their clients wait for any chemotherapy or radiation treatment (both of which can be either very toxic to the body or cause inherent health hazards) until after alternative therapies have had a chance at success... .

The goal of alternative therapy is to strengthen the body's immune system. These therapies may include treatments that rely on biopharmaceutical, immune enhancement, metabolic, nutritional, and herbal nontoxic methods.

代替療法医

固有の健康ハザード

生物薬剤的，免疫学的増強，薬草非毒性

〔出典 C, p.94：L25 〜 p.96：R27（一部抜粋）〕

(6) Alternative therapy

To make sure of your reading

Pick up pluses and minuses of each treatment for cancer.

The Lymphatic System

医学英語の常識（5）
語源と医学英語：cancer（癌）はなぜ蟹？

　医学英語は英語ではない，という人がいるのは，それらのほとんどがラテン語，ギリシア語を語源とする英語であるために見慣れないからであろう．また，日常使う英語でも，ラテン語やギリシア語に由来する語が多いのである．

　たとえば cancer はドイツ語で Krebs，フランス語で cancer といい，癌を意味すると同時にすべて"蟹座または蟹"という意味で用いられる．英語の cancer はラテン語に由来し，それはギリシア語の karkinos（＝蟹）を語源としている．医学の祖ヒポクラテス（Hippocrates：460?-?377B.C.）が乳癌の患者の乳房を切り開いた時，癌腫がまるで蟹の甲羅のようであり，その周囲の静脈が蟹が足を広げているように見え，そうよんだことから癌の意味で用いられた．英語の carcinoma は，karkinos により近い語である．また，tumor，growth も癌の意味に用いられ，malignant tumor，malignant growth というと悪性腫瘍を意味する．

　たとえば，血液の癌，白血病 leukemia は，leukos（ギリシア語＝ white），haima（ギリシア語＝ blood），-ia（ギリシア語，ラテン語＝病気の状態）が語源である．造血器の進行性悪性疾患で，血液・骨髄中に白血球およびその芽球が異常に増加するのが特徴である．cardiology は cardium が心臓，logos が言葉から学問の意味となった．よって，心臓学を指す．たとえば schizophrenia は，skhizō が裂ける，phrēn が仕切り・精神なので，精神が分裂した状態（統合失調症）を意味する．diaphragm は dia-（横切る），phrēn が横隔膜．respiration は，re- が再び，spirit は呼吸，あるいは魂．古代の人々にとっては，生きているということは呼吸していることであるから，それは横隔膜のあたりに魂が存在しており，人は死ぬと息をしなくなるのは，魂が外に出てしまうこと……であった．すべての医学英語学習の際に語源をたどっていると時間がかかるが，ときにはこのような言葉の旅をして楽しむのもいかがかと思う．

医学英語のルーツ―ギリシア神話（4）
モルヒネは眠りの神ヒュピノスの息子モルペウスから，麻薬中毒は自己愛者ナルキッソスから

　あら，皆さん，こっくりこ，こっくりこ……．ヒュピノス（Hypnos）[1]が木の枝であなた方の額にそうっと触れたようだ．ヒュピノスは夜の神ニュクスの息子，眠りの神様．常夜の国に近い山奥の洞窟のもっとも奥深い場所にある広い部屋で，ベッドは象牙，ふわふわと柔らかい毛に覆われたマットに，黒っぽいカバーを被って，今の皆さんと同じようにうとうと……と眠っている．そして息子の夢の神モルペウス（Morpheus）[2]が翼をひろげて周りを飛びながら父親の眠りを見守っている．そこには芥子や蓮などの花々が咲き乱れる薬草園があるそうな．

　ヒュピノスには，大きくひらひらした耳と翼があり，手には眠りの象徴であるけしの実をもっている．けしの実からは，そう，アヘン（opium）が抽出される．大昔から人々はその未熟果実に切り目を入れて，乳状の果汁をしぼり乾燥させたアヘンを鎮痛薬として用いたのである．

　アヘンに含まれるモルヒネをアルカロイド（alkaloid）[3]として初めて抽出したのは1805年，北ドイツの町の薬局助手，ゼルチュルネル（F.W.A. Sertürner：1783-1841）による．その化学物質をモルペウス（Morpheus）にちなんでモルヒネ（Morphin）と命名したのである．それが皮下注射として実用に至ったのは1853年のことであった．現在，このモルヒネのおかげで，がん患者の痛みは軽減されるようになってきた．夜ごと優しい眠りをもたらすヒュピノスとその息子モルペウスに感謝しよう．でも皆さんはこっくりこしないで！　まだ続きがあるのです．

　眠りには，突然睡魔に襲われるナルコレプシー（narcolepsy）という遺伝性の難病がある．患者は，昼間の睡眠発作や情動性脱力感だけでなく，入眠時の幻覚，夜間の呼吸困難に終生悩まされる．

　さて，ナルコレプシーという症状名はギリシア神話に登場する超イケメンのナルキッソス（Narkissos）に由来する．美しい彼に，ひとりのニンフが恋した．「こんにちはー」「あそぼー」と声をかけるがナルキッソスは知らん顔．戻ってくるのは自分の声ばかり．とうとう木霊（echo）になってしまっ

たという．

　ある日，泉にやってきた彼は水を飲もうとした．すると，水面にひとりの美しいオノコがいるではないか．彼は一目惚れしてしまった．毎日，毎日，泉に来てオノコを抱こうとするがすぐに姿が崩れてしまう．とうとう苦しみのあまり水辺で死んでしまった．けれども彼の身勝手な仕打ちに憤慨していたエーコーの女友達は，もともと心根が優しい．彼の死を憐れんでその屍を水辺に葬ったのである．するとその場所に花が咲き，人々は Narkissos（和名は水仙．ギリシア神話では死の花といわれる）と名づけたのであった．

　やがて，自己愛を Narcissism，自己愛者を Narcissist とよぶようになった．これらの語は narke（麻痺）に由来する．確かに水仙の花は強い香気を放ち，しかも葉は有毒であるし，とくに球根にも神経麻痺物質が含有されているそうだ．誰しも自分を愛しているもの．しかし malignant narcissism（悪性自己愛）はいただけない．

　さて，人生には時折落とし穴があるもの．居眠りがすぎて科目履修不可となるのも人生の落とし穴．もっと大きな穴は，人を"ハイ"な快感を覚えさせるアヘン，モルヒネ，コカイン（cocaine）などの麻薬中毒（narcotism）なのだ……．

注
1) ヒュピノスは，ローマ神話におけるソムヌス（Somnus）に相当する．cf. 不眠症：insomnia
2) モルペウスはヒュプノスと同一視されることがある．「夢」には複数の神々がいて役割が異なる．オネイロス（Oneiros）も「夢」であり，医学英語では 連結系 oneir- が以下のように夢に関するいくつかの用語をつくる．
3) アルカロイドには，モルヒネのほかにニコチン，コカイン，キニーネ，カフェイン，エフェドリン，クラーレがある．

眠りの神々と自己愛者ナルキッソスに因む医学英語

echocardiography　心エコー検査（法）
hypnogenic　催眠薬

hypnopompic hallucination　覚醒時幻覚（narcolepsyで見られる）
morphine　モルヒネ
morphinism　モルヒネ中毒
narcotics　麻酔薬
narcomania, narcotism　麻薬中毒
oneirocriticism　夢判断
oneirology　夢解釈学
oneirophrenia　夢幻精神病

CHAPTER 6
The Respiratory System　呼吸器系

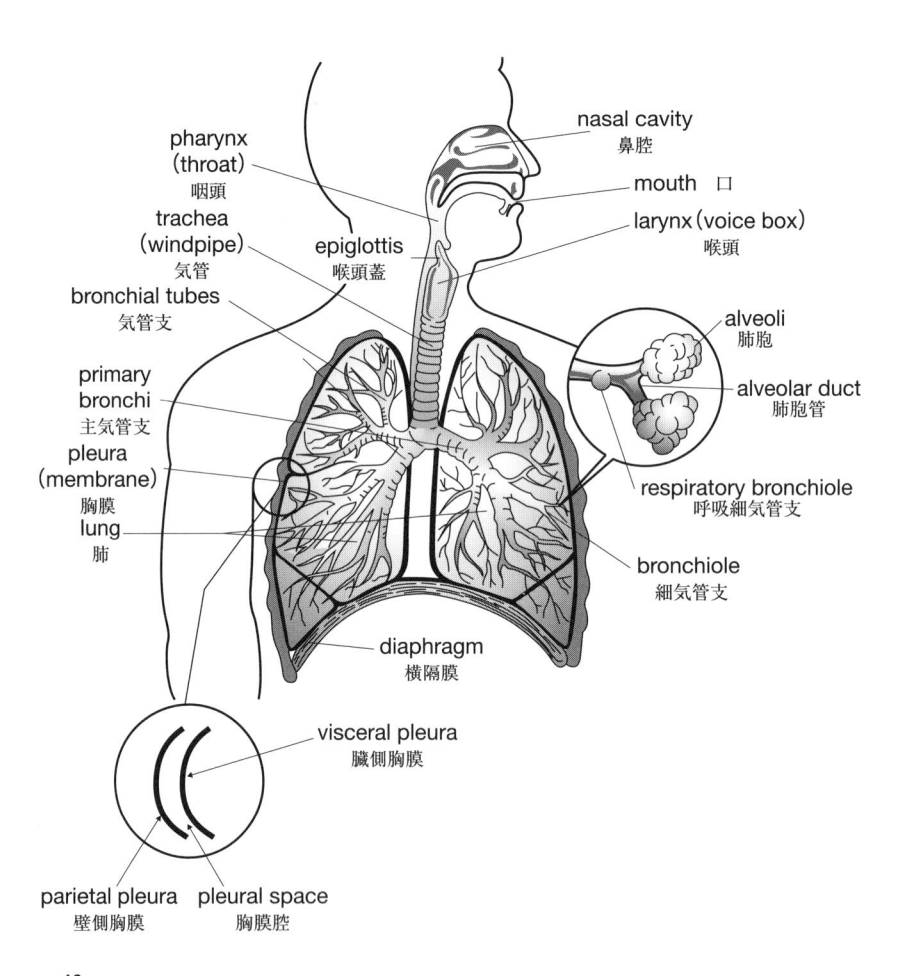

- pharynx (throat) 咽頭
- nasal cavity 鼻腔
- mouth 口
- trachea (windpipe) 気管
- larynx (voice box) 喉頭
- epiglottis 喉頭蓋
- bronchial tubes 気管支
- alveoli 肺胞
- primary bronchi 主気管支
- alveolar duct 肺胞管
- pleura (membrane) 胸膜
- respiratory bronchiole 呼吸細気管支
- lung 肺
- bronchiole 細気管支
- diaphragm 横隔膜
- visceral pleura 臟側胸膜
- parietal pleura 壁側胸膜
- pleural space 胸膜腔

Background Information

The lungs are cone-shaped organs, large enough to fill the pleural portion of the thoracic cavity completely. They extend from the diaphragm to a point slightly above the clavicles and lie against the ribs both anteriorly and posteriorly. The medial surface of each lung is roughly concave to allow room for the mediastinal structures[1] and for the heart, but concavity is greater on the left than on the right because of the position of the heart.

胸腔．体腔は Appendix. 参照．

縦隔構造，凹面

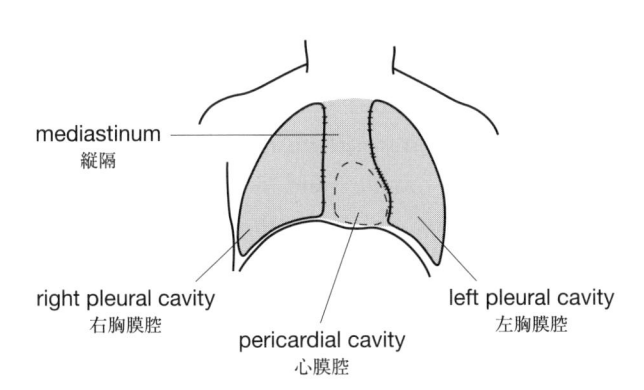

mediastinum
縦隔

right pleural cavity
右胸膜腔

pericardial cavity
心膜腔

left pleural cavity
左胸膜腔

The primary bronchi and pulmonary blood vessels (bound together by connective tissue to form what is known as the *root* of the lung) enter each lung through a slit on its medial surface called the *hilum*. The broad inferior surface of the lung, which rests on

第一次気管支

肺根

（肺）門

The Respiratory System

the diaphragm, constitutes the *base*, whereas the pointed upper margin is the *apex*.   肺底 / 肺尖

The left lung is partially divided by fissures into two *lobes*(upper and lower) and the right lung into three lobes(upper, middle, and lower).   葉

Visceral pleura[2] covers the outer surfaces of the lungs and adheres to them much as the skin of an apple adheres to the apple.   臓側胸膜 / 付着する

Alveoli and other respiratory tubes ― 肺胞と呼吸器官

Oxygen is needed by cells to use (burn) in order to produce heat and energy.   In using the oxygen, carbon dioxide is produced and the respiratory system disposes of it and other gases.   The exchange of oxygen for carbon dioxide within the lungs is called respiration[3].   The action of inhaling and exhaling, called breathing, is carried on by the ribs, rib muscles, and diaphragm.   When the rib muscles and diaphragm contract, air rushes into the lungs; when they relax, air is forced out by the change of lung size and pressure within the lung and chest cavity.   吸息, 呼息 / 横隔膜

The upper respiratory tract includes the following: the nose with nostrils, mouth, throat, and the larynx, plus numerous sinus (cavities) within the head.   Inhaled air is filtered, moistened, and warmed as it is passed through the larynx or voice box containing the vocal cords.   The "clean, filtered air" passes on into the lower respiratory tract, which includes the following: the trachea or windpipe, bronchi, and the lungs, which contain bronchial tubes and alveoli or air sacs... .   One bronchus goes to the left lung and one to the   洞（単複同形）/ 声帯 / 気管支

Alveoli and other respiratory tubes

right lung. Within the lungs the bronchi divide into smaller branches called bronchial tubes.

At the ends of these tubes there are tiny clusters of minute air sacs called alveoli.

The function of alveoli — in fact, the function of the entire respiratory system — is to bring air close enough to blood for oxygen to get into the blood and carbon dioxide to get out of it. Two facts about the structure of alveoli make them able to perform this function admirably. First, the wall of each alveolus is made up of a single layer of cells and so are the walls of the capillaries around it. This means that between the blood in the capillaries and the air in the alveolus there is a barrier probably less than 1/5,000 of an inch thick! Second, there are millions of alveoli. This means that together they make an enormous surface (in the neighborhood of 1,100 square feet, an area many times larger than the surface of the entire body) where large amounts of oxygen and carbon dioxide can rapidly be exchanged.

> 房
> 単数形 alveolus,〔出典 A, p.v：L30 〜 R.5〕
>
> one over five thousand
>
> 約, 平方フィート

注

1) mediastinal structure = mediastinum　縦隔構造：左右の肺に挟まれた中央部. 胸腺, 大動脈弓, 心膜, 種々の神経・神経叢, 気管, 食道, 胸管, リンパ管, リンパ節などが収まっている.

2) visceral pleura　臓側胸膜（肺胸膜）：肺と肺葉溝の表面を覆う. parietal pleura　壁側胸膜（肺腔壁の各部分：肋骨, 横隔膜, 縦隔を裏打ちする）.

3) respiration = re-（接頭辞：反復）+ spir-（連結形：呼吸）+ -ation（接尾辞：動作の意）. spirit は元来, ラテン語で息の意味から, 後に「精神」の意味で使用されるようになった.

The Respiratory System

Let's pronounce medical English terms.

1. alveoli 2. bronchus 3. trachea
4. diaphragm 5. carbon dioxide

Review questions

1. How many lobes does each lung have?
2. What is there between two lungs?
3. What surrounds around each lobe?
4. What function does the lung perform?
5. Select the appropriate definition for each word.
   1) alveoli   (   )   2) respiration (   )
   3) bronchus   (   )   4) diaphragm   (   )
   5) lungs   (   )
   a. the grape-like tiny sacs where gas exchanges take place
   b. either of the two organs in chest that you use for respiration
   c. repeating actions of inhaling and exhaling
   d. any of the major passages into the lungs
   e. a domelike and muscular partition that controls the size of the chest cavity
6. Write the medical English for each daily English word used daily.
   1) breathing (   )
   2) windpipe   (   )
   3) voice box (   )

Supplementary Reading

The Sea and Poison（海と毒薬）

作者：遠藤周作（1923-1996），**作品出版年**：1958
あらすじ：第二次世界大戦中，北九州で日本軍に撃ち落とされたアメリカ軍B29の捕虜に生体解剖手術が行われた．その事実を小説化した遠藤周作の『海と毒薬』の英訳 "The Sea and Poison" からの抜粋．

　肺をどこまで切除すると人間は死ぬかという生体解剖（vivisection）が行われる場面には，執刀医おやじ（次期医学部長の座をめざす橋本教授，英文では The Old Man）と柴田助教授，第一助手の浅井，そしてインターンの戸田，勝呂、主任看護師大場，看護師，見学者の軍医，将校たちが登場する．

　描写の中心は，悪に無感覚な戸田と，心の中に起きる葛藤に耐えかねる勝呂との対比であるといえよう．作者は，登場人物に現代の私たち日本人を重ね合わせることで人間の普遍性を暗示するとともに，この人体実験は今，どこでも日常的に起こりうることを示唆していると考えられる〔出典 D〕.

　The Old Man and Dr Shibata appeared at three o'clock, dressed in surgical gowns, their faces half-hidden by their masks.　They were surrounded by the officers.　The Old Man stopped for an instant at the threshold and glanced at Suguro, who was still leaning against the wall on the verge of weeping.　Then he quickly looked away and walked in. ...

　"What's today?" Breaking in, the short fat medical officer who had left the 'bounty' in Dr Shibata's room made a gesture with his finger on his shaven head. "Are you going to cut here?"

　"No, no lobotomy.　Tomorrow Doctor Kondo and

おやじ（橋本教授）
手術着

敷居（入口）
泣き出さんばかりに

口をはさむ
誉（タバコの名称）

脳の白質切開術

The Respiratory System

Doctor Arajima are going to perform that sort of experiment on another prisoner."

"Then with you it's just the lung?"

"Yes, sir."...

The figure of the prisoner lying with his face towards the ceiling differed in no way from that of ordinary patients. The prickly sensation of being about to murder someone did not stir at all in Toda. He felt that all would be brought automatically to a proper conclusion. With a certain sluggishness, he inserted the long, thin catheter tube into the prisoner's nostrils. The nose was long with a reddish tip, the nose of a white man. All Toda had to do was to adjust the nozzle of the oxygen machine to complete the preparations. The ether seemed to have taken full effect. The prisoner was sleeping, a slight snore coming through the tube. Thick leather straps firmly bound his legs in the green fatigue trousers and both his hands. Oblivious to the gaze of those around him, he faced upwards toward the ceiling. This expression was so relaxed that it looked almost as though a faint smile were playing about his lips.

"We should get started, eh, Doctor?" Dr Shibata asked the Old Man after checking the blood pressure gauge. The Old Man, who had been staring at the floor, gave a start as he heard the question. ...

"The vivisection is beginning at 3 : 08 pm. Toda, put that in the record."

The Old Man took the electric scalpel in his hand and bent over the prisoner. Toda could hear the dull whir of the movie camera behind him. Dr Araji-

ちくちくする痛み

カテーテル〔kæθ(ə)tər〕
鼻孔

いびき

…知らないで

唇のあたりにただよう

血圧計〔géidʒ〕

記録する
電動メス

ma of Second Surgery had started to record the vivisection process.

......

"Scalpel."

"Gauze." ガーゼ〔gɔ́ːz〕

"Scalpel."

Dr Shibata directed Chief Nurse Oba in a hoarse voice.

"Next," Suguro thought, "it'll be the raspatory and 骨膜剥離器
cutting the rib bone." 肋骨

As an intern, he could tell just from Dr Shibata's commands where the Old Man was cutting on the prisoner's body and could picture exactly what was occurring.

Suguro shut his eyes. He shut his eyes and tried to think that he was not really involved in a vivisection being performed on a prisoner but that this was a routine operation performed on a regular patient. ... いつもの手術

But then there was the dull sound of a rib bone snapping and, a moment later, the lighter sound of it dropping into the receptacle echoing from the walls of the operating theatre. The ether had been cut off perhaps. The prisoner suddenly let out a low pitched groan.

The pounding in Suguro's chest, the whispering within him increased in tempo: "To help, to help!"...

At that moment Asai's voice echoed sharply; 'The prisoner's left lung has been removed entirely. Now the excision of the upper section of the right lung is in process. In experiments performed up to now, when half of both lungs together have been excised,

The Respiratory System

the result has been instant death.'...

"Forty......thirty-five......thirty." Toda was reading the blood pressure gauge. "Thirty......twenty-five......twenty......fifteen......ten. That's it. It's over."

After he had relayed this information to the Old Man and Dr Shibata as his job demanded, Toda slowly straightened up. ...

"So it's done!" The fat medical officer standing in the front row wiped the sweat from his head with a handkerchief. "What was the time?"

"4 : 28," Asai answered. "The operation began at 3 : 08; therefore the time taken was one hour and twenty minutes."

The Old Man looked down at the corpse, not saying a word. His gloved hands, gleaming with smeared blood under the ceiling light, still tightly gripped the scalpel. As though to thrust him out of the way, Chief Nurse Oba pushed herself between him and the table and covered the corpse with a white sheet. Staggering slightly, the Old Man retreated two or three steps, but he still just stood there, without making a move.

死体
血で汚れて光っている

注) vivisection（生体解剖）= vivi-（連結形）+ section（語根）:"解剖の行為・切開・剥離すること"を英語では dissection といい,"生きた・生体の"という意味の連結形の vivi- が結合して vivisection という単語となった.

人間の循環器系は心臓と肺と血液であるが，肺は呼吸と血液浄化作用を行う器官である．体中からの CO_2 を含んだ血液は，小さな肺胞のまわりにまとわりついた細い細い（直径約 7 μm の赤血球でさえ一列にならなければ通れないほど細い）血管にまでたどりつき，肺胞へと入る．そこで炭酸ガスと酸素の交換がすばやく行われ，新鮮な血液は心臓へと戻っていく．

To make sure of your reading

What's the difference between the attitude of two interns, Toda and Suguro? Pick up the English expressions to give the evidence of your idea.

The Respiratory System

医学英語の常識 (6)
新型インフルエンザ

2009年春頃から2010年3月にかけ，Influenza A virus subtype H1N1（A型H1N1亜型）というインフルエンザ（流行性感冒）が世界的に流行した．以下の記事から医学英語を学習しよう〔出典E〕．

The 2009 flu pandemic was a global outbreak of a new strain of H1N1 influenza virus, often referred to as "swine flu". First described in April 2009, the virus appeared to be a new strain of H1N1 which resulted when a previous triple reassortment of bird, pig, and human flu viruses further combined with a Eurasian pig flu virus. Unlike most strains of influenza, H1N1 does not disproportionately infect adults older than 60 years; this was an unusual and characteristic feature of the H1N1 pandemic. Even for persons previously very healthy, a small percentage of patients will develop viral pneumonia or acute respiratory distress syndrome. This manifests itself as increased breathing difficulty and typically occurs 3-6 days after initial onset of flu symptoms.

問
1. 新型インフルエンザを英語でどういうか？
2. the flu pandemicには定冠詞theがあり，influenzaには冠詞がないのはなぜか？
3. H1N1 influenzaのH1N1のフルスペリングは？
4. なぜswine fluというのか？
5. the pandemicを日本語ではどういうか？

では，少し詳細に説明しながら答えよう．

答
1. 新型インフルエンザは，以下のようによばれる．
   a. the flu pandemic
   b. H1N1 influenza（H1N1型インフルエンザ）

= Influenza A virus subtype H1N1（A型H1N1亜型インフルエンザ）
　c. swine flu（豚インフルエンザ）
　d. a new influenza（新型インフルエンザ），A/H1N1 pdm（A型H1N1型流行性感冒），pdm = pandemic
2. viral pneumonia（肺炎），acute respiratory distress syndrome（急性呼吸器窮迫症候群）のように，通常，病名には冠詞は不要．fluはすべての急性ウイルス感染を含む病態を表わすので，influenzaの省略語では，特定するtheを必要とする．病名と冠詞についてはp.84を参照のこと．
3. H = hemagglutinin（赤血球凝集素）．抗体のように血球凝集を起こす．N = neuraminidase（ノイラミニダーゼ= sialidase シアリダーゼ：酵素）．ウイルスや細菌，原虫由来の微生物，脊椎動物の各種組織に存在する．オリゴ糖類，糖タンパク，糖脂質から末端のアセチルノイラミン酸残基への加水分解を触媒する．数字の1はタイプの分類記号．
4. 脊椎動物のブタの組織に存在し，あるいはウイルスがブタを介して人に感染するため．しかし，ユダヤ教では豚を食べることが禁じられているので，イスラエルの保健副大臣は2009年4月28日，「メキシコ・インフルエンザ」という呼称を用いると発表した．病名も文化によって異なることに注意．
5. 「汎発性流行病」「世界的流行病」という．
　pan- すべての + demo- 人々．Gk：demos = people.
　epi-（pref）上の + demos = epidemic「流行病」
　en- 中の，内の + demos = endemic「地方病・風土病」

そのほかに知っておいてほしいこと

1. influenzaの語源：（18世紀初出）ラテン語のinfluentialから．インフルエンザは星の影響（influence）によると考えられたことから．
2. vaccine〔vǽksiːn〕ワクチン．語源はラテン語vacca = cow（雌牛）．
3. virus〔váɪərəs〕= L. slimy liquid（粘着性液体）

CHAPTER 7
The Digestive System　消化器系

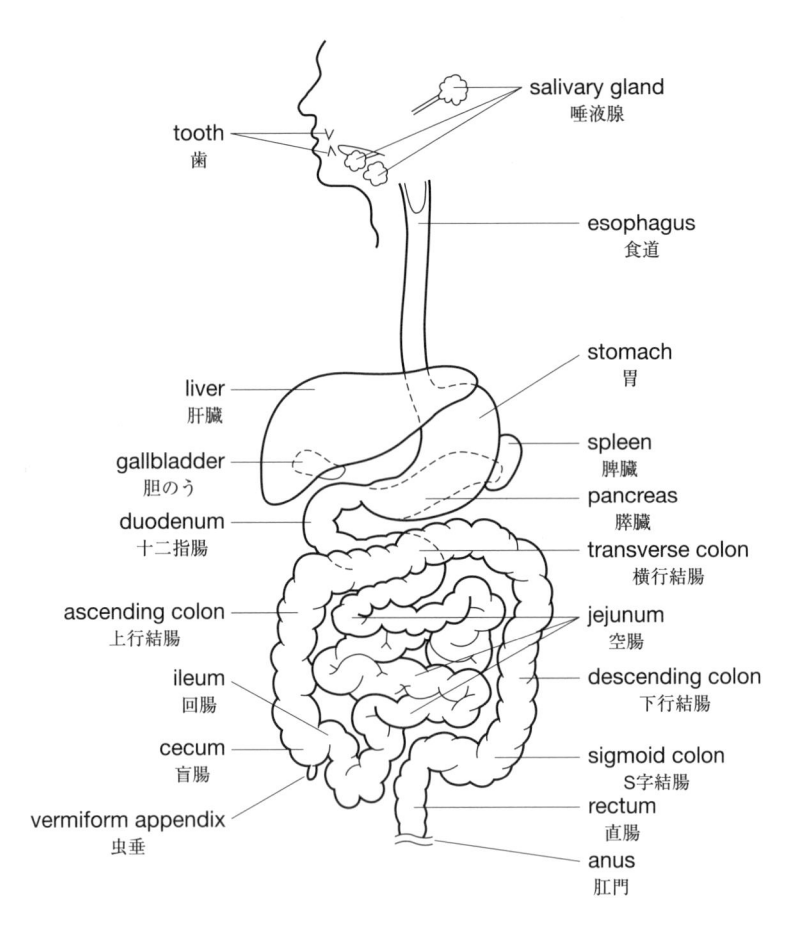

- tooth　歯
- salivary gland　唾液腺
- esophagus　食道
- stomach　胃
- liver　肝臓
- spleen　脾臓
- gallbladder　胆のう
- pancreas　膵臓
- duodenum　十二指腸
- transverse colon　横行結腸
- ascending colon　上行結腸
- jejunum　空腸
- ileum　回腸
- descending colon　下行結腸
- cecum　盲腸
- sigmoid colon　S字結腸
- vermiform appendix　虫垂
- rectum　直腸
- anus　肛門

The main digestive organs 主要消化器官
(1) Teeth and salivary glands — 歯, 唾液腺

The teeth function to hold, tear, and masticate the food. The small pieces are moved around by the tongue, and the chewing process allows the food to become thoroughly mixed with saliva. There are three pairs of salivary glands that open into the mouth cavity. These are the parotid, submaxillary, and the sublingual. Their secretions not only moisten the food to aid in swallowing, but also add an enzyme which begins the conversion of starches to sugar. The tongue moves the food mass to the rear of the mouth where the food is swallowed.

咀嚼する

唾液〔səláɪvə〕

耳下腺, 顎下腺
舌下腺
嚥下, 酵素

Oral cavity — 口腔

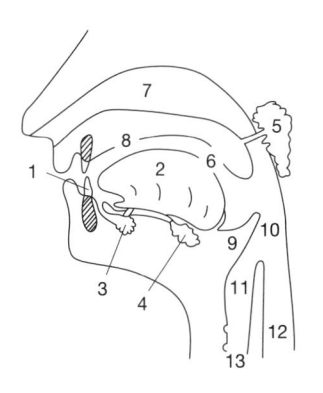

1. tooth　歯
2. tongue　舌
3. sublingual gland　舌下腺
4. submaxillary gland　顎下腺
5. parotid gland　耳下腺
6. oral cavity　口腔
7. nasal cavity　鼻腔
8. palate　口蓋
9. epiglottis　喉頭蓋
10. pharynx　咽頭
11. larynx　喉頭
12. esophagus　食道
13. trachea　気管

The Digestive System

Tooth ― 歯

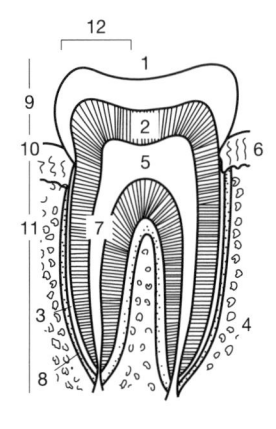

1. enamel　エナメル
2. dentine　象牙質
3. cementum　セメント質
4. bone　骨
5. pulp cavity　歯髄腔
6. gingiva (gum)　歯肉（発音注意）
7. root canal　歯根管
8. peridontal membrane　歯根膜
9. crown　歯冠
10. neck　頸部
11. root　歯根
12. cusp　尖頭

(2) Esophagus and stomach ― 食道と胃

A muscular tube, the esophagus, which is about 25 to 30 cm long and 2.5 cm in diameter, receives the food mass and moves it along to the stomach. This is accomplished by a wave of muscular contractions (peristalsis) which forces the food downward. The cardiac valve controls the entrance of food into the stomach.

〔daɪǽmətər〕

蠕動

The stomach is a muscular sac lined with a mucous membrane. It receives the food and adds gastric juices (enzymes and hydrochloric acid). As the food is churned by this muscular organ, chemical reactions take place which reduce the more complex proteins into simpler substances.

胃液
塩酸

Stomach — 胃

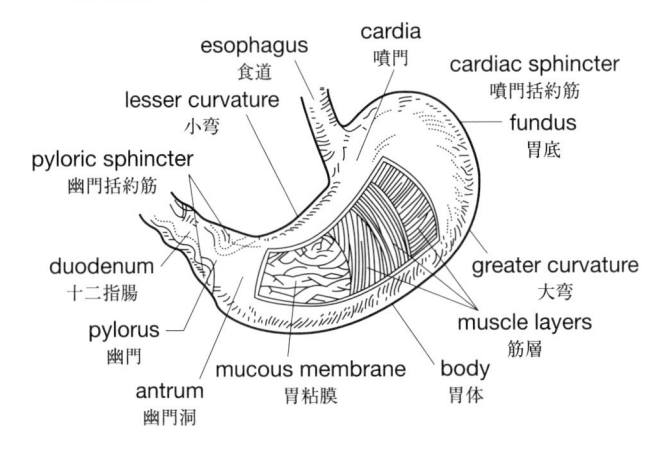

- esophagus 食道
- cardia 噴門
- cardiac sphincter 噴門括約筋
- lesser curvature 小弯
- fundus 胃底
- pyloric sphincter 幽門括約筋
- duodenum 十二指腸
- pylorus 幽門
- antrum 幽門洞
- mucous membrane 胃粘膜
- body 胃体
- greater curvature 大弯
- muscle layers 筋層

(3) Small intestine —小腸

The pyloric valve controls the release of the partially digested food material into the small intestine. This organ is about six to nine meters in length and about 2.5 cm in diameter.　It has three main divisions: duodenum, jejunum, and ileum.　The digestive juices of the liver, gallbladder, and the pancreas are added near the junction of the stomach and the duodenum.　The digestive process is continued and complex proteins, carbohydrates, and fats reduced to simpler forms more easily absorbed.　Small finger-like projections (villi) of the inner surface of the small intestine greatly increases the absorptive[1] surface area. The absorbed food material is taken up by blood vessels to be transported to all body parts.

括約筋弁

タンパク質，炭水化物

絨毛〔vílai〕

吸収する

注）absorptive は名詞 absorption の形容詞形（名詞形 absorption は動詞 absorb と綴りが異なることに注意）．

The Digestive System

Inside of the small intestine ― 小腸内部構造

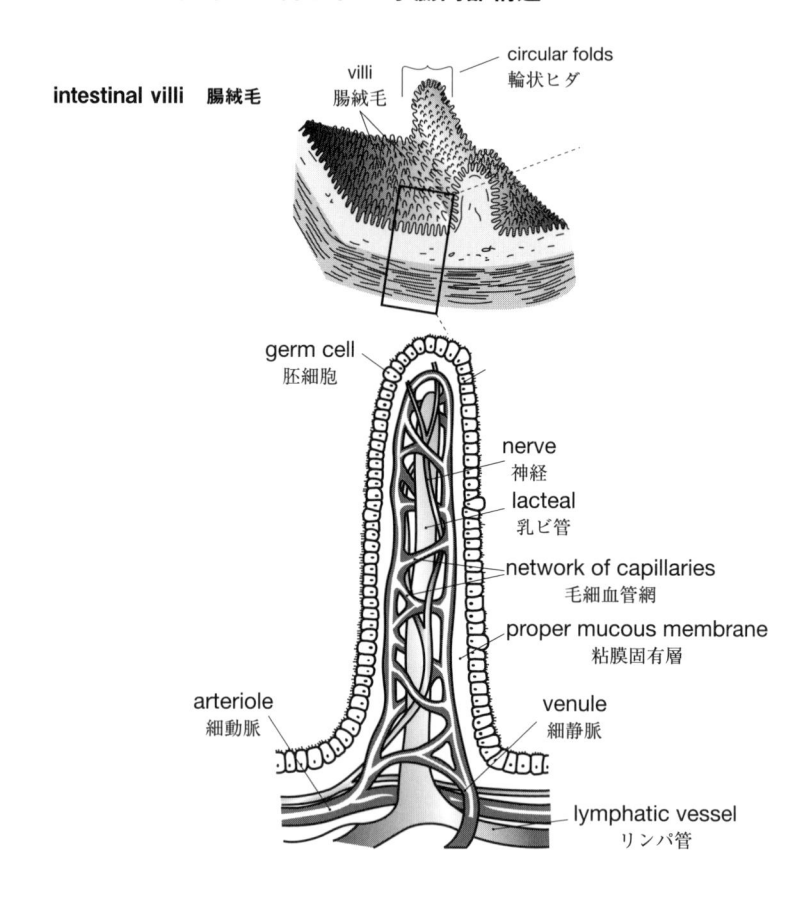

intestinal villi　腸絨毛

villi
腸絨毛

circular folds
輪状ヒダ

germ cell
胚細胞

nerve
神経

lacteal
乳ビ管

network of capillaries
毛細血管網

proper mucous membrane
粘膜固有層

arteriole
細動脈

venule
細静脈

lymphatic vessel
リンパ管

(4) Large intestine ―大腸

The remaining material is moved to the large intestine. This organ is 1.5 to 2.5 meters in length and may be 5 to 7.5 cm in diameter. Its main function is to consolidate the wastes by removing water. The rectum is a section of the tube between the large intestine and the external opening of the tract (anus).

硬くする

(4) Large intestine

It functions to control the release of solid wastes.

〔出典 A, p.v : R25 ～ p. vi : L14〕

Let's pronounce medical English terms.

1. peristalsis   2. salivary gland   3. esophagus
4. stomach   5. villus   6. pylorus
7. duodenum   8. anus

Review questions

1. With what juice is the food mixed in the stomach?
2. Give the names of the divisions which compose of the small intestine.
3. Give the names of the divisions which compose of the large intestine.
4. Select the appropriate word for each phrases.
   1) numerous small projections of the lining of the small intestine (　　)
   2) the product that are no longer needed and are expel from the body (　　)
   3) the muscular organ where the food is churned with chemical substances and change it to small pieces (　　)
   4) the muscular contractions which push the content to the next organ forward, creating wavelike movements (　　)
   5) the digestive juice secreted membrane of the stomach to promote digestion (　　)
   a. stomach   b. peristalsis   c. waste
   d. gastric juice e. villi
5. Select the word or phrases related to each word(s).
   1) salivary glands   (　　)
   2) stomach   (　　)
   3) pancreas   (　　)
   4) large intestine   (　　)
   5) peristalsis   (　　)
   a. a fingerlike structure
   b. pass food from mouth to stomach
   c. waste product with little water
   d. wormlike movement

The Digestive System

    e. villi
    f. large gland to the duodenum
    g. hydrochloric acid
    h. three glands

The accessory digestive organs　付属消化器官
Liver and gallbladder — 肝臓・胆のう

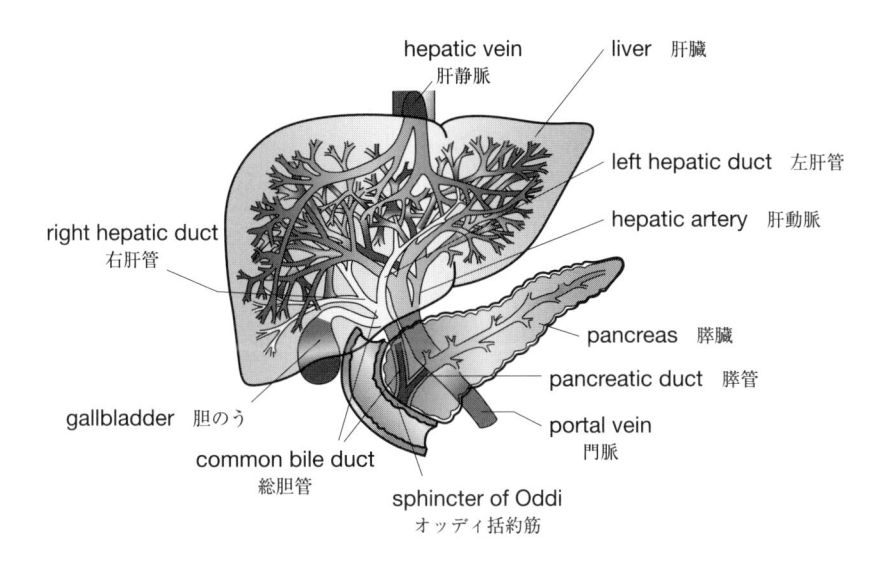

- hepatic vein　肝静脈
- liver　肝臓
- left hepatic duct　左肝管
- hepatic artery　肝動脈
- right hepatic duct　右肝管
- pancreas　膵臓
- pancreatic duct　膵管
- gallbladder　胆のう
- portal vein　門脈
- common bile duct　総胆管
- sphincter of Oddi　オッディ括約筋

Background Information

The liver, like the salivary glands and pancreas, is an outgrowth of the digestive tube: it is a very large gland opening off the beginning of the small intestine (*duodenum*). In the embryo it is at first a mid-line organ, but its right side soon outpaces the left. At birth, three quarters of the liver is to the right of the mid-line, and in an adult, seven eighths. The liver completely fills the part of the abdomen that is covered by the right side of the diaphragm and rib-cage.

All the blood from the spleen and from the stomach and intestine is passed to the liver by the *portal vein*. It seeps through the substance of the liver and

唾液腺
生成器官

十二指腸、胚
…をしのぐ
3/4
7/8

肋骨籠

浸透する

The Digestive System

returns to the general circulation by way of the *inferior vena cava*.　　下（行）大静脈
In the process the liver cells take up materials digested and absorbed from the food.

The blood from the portal vein is the raw material on which the liver works. In addition, fresh blood is supplied by the *hepatic artery*.　　肝動脈

The digestive secretion of the liver, the *bile*, flows through small channels to the common bile duct,　　総胆管
which opens into the duodenum. Bile is formed continuously but is most needed when there is a meal to be digested. Between meals most of it is stored in the *gallbladder*, a bag projecting from the cystic (bile)　　胆のう
duct and stuck to the underside of the liver, able to contract and eject bile when stimulated by food in the　　排出する，刺激される
duodenum.

The liver is an organ of *digestion*, and of *excretion*.　　排泄
Its many other functions include *synthesis* of proteins　　合成
and other substances needed elsewhere, such as glu-　　〔glú:kous〕
cose, amino-acids, and the proteins of the blood; *stor-*　　アミノ酸，貯蔵
age, especially of glucose (in the form of *glycogen*); and
neutralization of poisons. These are functions of liv-　　中和
ing cells in general, but many of the tissues of the body have become so specialized that they are no longer self-supporting in these respects. In several ways the liver is essential to life. The most urgent is keeping a steady concentration of glucose in the blood to replace what is consumed as fuel. The brain keeps no stores at all, and quickly dies if supplies from the liver are cut off.

Let's pronounce medical English terms.

1. liver   2. gallbladder   3. portal vein
4. bile   5. glycogen

Review questions

1. What is the digestive secretion of the liver?
2. Explain the functions of the liver.
3. Select the appropriate definition for each word.
   1) common bile duct   (   )
   2) liver   (   )
   3) gallbladder   (   )
   4) portal vein   (   )
   5) glycogen   (   )
   a. the large gland in the top of the abdomen on the right side of the body, involved in many metabolic processes
   b. the sac situated underneath the liver, in which bile is stored
   c. a vessel carrying blood to the liver from the stomach, pancreas, intestine, and the spleen
   d. a form of substance change from glucose by the action of insulin, and stored in the liver
   e. a tube where the common hepatic duct joins the bile duct and carries bile to the duodenum

The Digestive System

医学英語の常識（7）
病名と冠詞

　通常，器官名は定冠詞 the を必要とし，病名には冠詞が不要である．しかし，何事にも例外があるように，病名にも冠詞を必要とする場合がある．以下にいくつかの例を病名を含む簡単な英文によって示す．

（1）a（症状を表わす）
I have a cold.
You have a fever.
My mother has a headache.（toothache, stomachache）
I have a sore throat.（のどがひりひりする）
A VIP（very important person）like a company president tends to have a heart attack.（VIP をビップと読むと侮蔑的になるので要注意）
My baby has a rash.
I suffer from a runny nose every spring.
Do you have a stomachache?

（2）the（よく知られた病気）
My son has the mumps.（おたふく風邪）
My father has the sniffles.（鼻かぜ）
My child has the chicken pox.（水ぼうそう）
I used to have the hives in spring.（じんましん）
ただし，最近では冠詞を省略する傾向がある．

（3）無冠詞
It's a kind of stress.
My father died of lung cancer.
You have diabetes.
Who takes care of the woman who seems to have Alzheimer's disease?
I had asthma in my child days.

She suffers from constipation because of her sedentary work.
There's a lot of flu going around.（しばしば the flu）

The Digestive System

医学英語のルーツ―ギリシア神話（5）
接頭辞 epi- と pro- とプロメテウスの肝臓，そして pan- とパンドーラ

　巨神族ティターンはオリュンポスの神々に睨まれることをよくしでかす．エピメテウス（Epimetheus）とプロメテウス（Prometheus）兄弟もそうであった．このふたり，名前のごとくに性格が正反対なのだ．Epimetheus, Prometheus に共通する metheus の意味は「考える人（thinker）」，epi- は接頭辞で「上，追加，付属，外側」という意味であり，pro- は「前，公に」という意味である．というわけで Epimetheus は行動した後に考えるタイプ（after thinker）であり，よくいえばのんびりした性格．悪くいえば，「何とかのあと知恵」的であった．兄の Prometheus は事を起こすときに前もってよく考えるタイプ（fore thinker）である．よくいえば思慮分別があり，悪くいえば石橋を叩いて渡らない可能性がある．

　しかし，プロメテウスは行動力があり，正義感も強い，また考えることも大きい．人間を水と泥から創ったのも彼である．しかも暗闇で生活がうまくできない人間に同情して天の火を盗んで人間に与えた命知らずの，いや，命を惜しまない義者である．神々だけの特権であった火を人に与えたと知って，最高神のゼウスは烈火のごとく怒り猛ったことはいうまでもない．神罰としてプロメテウスはコーカサス山に鎖でつながれてしまった．雨，雷，風に吹き晒され，毎日ハゲワシが飛んできては彼の肝臓を食らうのだからたまったものではない．ところが，不思議なことにプロメテウスは死なないのだ．なぜだろう？

　人間ならば肝臓をすべて摘出すると 30 分で死ぬそうである．彼は巨神だから，その肝臓も巨大であっただろう．それに肝臓は増殖するものだから，ハゲワシの食べる程度では一晩で回復したと見える．となると，プロメテウスは終わりなき苦しみに耐えなければならない．しかし，捨てる神あれば，拾う神あり．神々の中で最大の英雄，ヘラクレス（Hercules）に助けられて彼は永遠の苦しみから解放された．われわれ人間を創り，火を与えてくれたプロメテウスは偉大であるけれど，ヘラクレスも負けず劣らず偉大である．

　彼らに比べるとエピメテウスには困ったものだ．ゼウスは彼の浅はかさに目をつけ，地上最初の女パンドーラ（Pandora）を彼の元に遣わした．彼女

の名は神々から「すべての（接頭辞：pan-）賜物を与えられた女（語根：dora）」という意味である．贈り物とはよきものばかりではない．パンドーラは表面は美しいが，心根は恥知らずでずるい女であった[1]．ゼウスの命令で，神々から「すべて」の贈り物が彼女に吹きこまれたからだ．

　エピメテウスは，愚かしくもなぜ女神のように美しい女が自分のもとにやって来たか，考えもしなかったようだ．一目見て「パンドーラ命」となった．でも，パンドーラはしばらくすると，勇気もなく，話に深みもない男に飽き飽きしてきたらしい．かといって恐いのは自分を人間への復讐のために遣わしたゼウス．鬱々として何か面白いことはないかしら？　と思案するうちに，「決して開いてはならんぞ」と戒められて持たされた甕を思い出した．戒めは破りたくなるものであるが，戒めには理由があるはず．考えもせずに開けてしまった．すると，なにやら怪しいもの―あらゆる災いと不幸が次から次へと，出てしまった．慌てふためいてふたりは蓋を閉めたが後の祭り……最後にかろうじて残ったのが「希望」だという．実体はないが，人の拠り所である希望が残されたのは神々のささやかな思いやりであろう．

　さて，同じく名前にpan-のつく女性に医術の神アスクレピウス（Aesculapius）の娘パナケイア（Panacea）がいる．目立たないが父を助けて医療に勤しみ，すべての病気を治療したといわれる．あなたはエピメテウスタイプ？　それともプロメテウスタイプ？　パンドーラタイプ，それともパナケイアタイプ？　どちらを目標にする？　いずれにしろ，あなたが学ぶ医療・医学のprofessionalになってほしい．

　そして，人体にはepi-（追加・後ろ・間）もpro-（前）もpan-もある（次頁参照）．

注）おそらく，このようなパンドーラの性質には当時，あるいは伝わった地域の女性に対する見方（偏見？）が込められている，と思われる．

The Digestive System

Prometheus, Epimetheus, Pandora に因む医学英語

epithelium　上皮細胞：epi- + thele（乳頭）+ ium（組織）．この細胞は乳頭だけでなく，血管のない層，皮膚，粘膜，膜漿，腺にある．

epinephrine　エピネフリン：副腎髄質ホルモン

prognosis　予後：pro- + gnosis（知識）．病気のたどる経過を前もって予測すること．あるいは告げること．

cf. diagnosis: dia- =完全に．患者を面談・診察・検査などによって病状を判断し，医学的結論をなすこと．患者の多種多様な背景が含まれる．

pancreas　膵臓：すべて肉（crea）のようなもの．他の臓器のように明確な被膜をもたない．

panacea　万能薬：Panacea は「ヒポクラテスの誓い」の冒頭で医神の父と他の姉妹とともに名をよばれる．

prostate　前立腺：ギリシア語で〜の前に立っている人．pro- + state（安定させる）

professional = pro- + fessio（= public declaration =公言）+ -al（=接尾辞=〜に関する）

CHAPTER 8
The Urinary System　泌尿器系

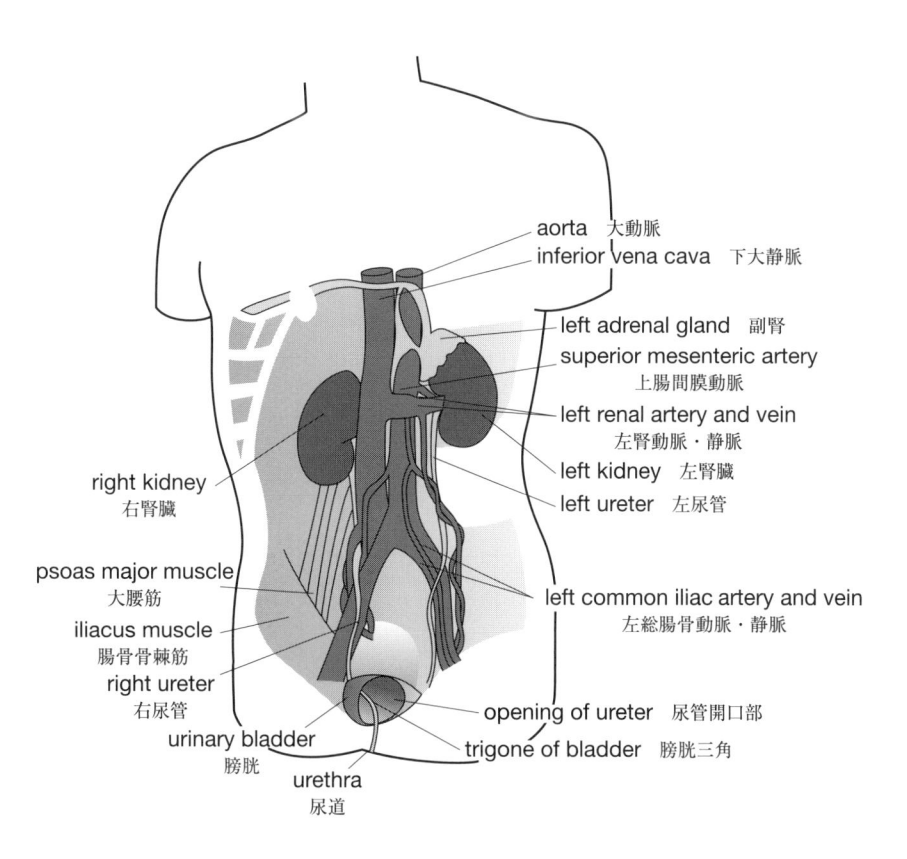

- aorta　大動脈
- inferior vena cava　下大静脈
- left adrenal gland　副腎
- superior mesenteric artery　上腸間膜動脈
- left renal artery and vein　左腎動脈・静脈
- left kidney　左腎臓
- left ureter　左尿管
- right kidney　右腎臓
- psoas major muscle　大腰筋
- iliacus muscle　腸骨骨棘筋
- right ureter　右尿管
- left common iliac artery and vein　左総腸骨動脈・静脈
- opening of ureter　尿管開口部
- urinary bladder　膀胱
- trigone of bladder　膀胱三角
- urethra　尿道

The Urinary System

Background Information

The urinary system, as you might guess from its name, performs the functions of secreting urine and eliminating it from the body. What you might not guess so easily is how essential these functions are for healthy survival. Unless the urinary system operates normally, the normal composition of blood cannot long be maintained, and serious consequences soon follow. In this chapter we shall discuss the structure and function of each of the urinary system's organs.

There are two kidneys. They lie behind the abdominal organs against the muscles of the back. Usually the left kidney is a little larger than the right and a little farther above the waistline. A heavy cushion of fat normally encases each kidney and helps hold it in place; so in a very thin person, the kidneys may drop down a little. This hinders urine drainage by putting a kink in the ureter, the tube that drains urine out of the kidneys.

The outer part of the kidney is called the *cortex*. (The word "cortex" comes from the Latin word that means bark or rind, so the cortex of an organ—the kidney, the brain, the adrenal glands—is its outer layer.) The interior part of the kidney, beneath the cortex, is the *medulla*.

Kidney cells and capillaries are arranged so that they form unique little structures called *nephrons*. Each nephron consists of three main parts: a glomerulus, a Bowman's capsule, and a tubule. The *glomerulus* is a network of blood capillaries tucked into the top of a microscopic-sized funnel shaped structure.

分泌すること
排泄すること

正常に動かない
成分
結果

ウエストライン
覆う，適所に

よじれ
尿

皮質

樹皮，外皮
副腎

髄質 [mədʌ́lə]

ネフロン（腎単位）
糸球体
ボーマン嚢 [báumən],
[kǽpsəl]
細管，漏斗型

Background Information

The top part of this structure is called *Bowman's capsule*, and the stem part is called the *renal tubule*. Different parts of the renal tubule have different names. The first segment of each tubule is called the proximal convoluted tubule—proximal because it lies nearest the tubule's origin from Bowman's capsule, and convoluted because it twists around to form several coils. The proximal convoluted tubule becomes the descending limb and then the ascending limb of the loop of Henle. The ascending limb becomes the distal convoluted tubule, which terminates in a straight, or collecting tubule that opens into the renal pelvis.

近位曲尿細管

起始点,回旋状

下行脚
ヘンレ係蹄, 遠位曲尿細管
腎盤

| Let's pronounce medical English terms. |

1. kidney　　2. nephron　　3. ureter
4. glomerulus　5. Bowman's capsule

| Review questions |

1. If the function of the urinary system failures, what happens?
2. What does the word 'cortex' mean in Latin?
3. What does the nephron consist of?
4. Find the appropriate definition for the following words.
   1) kidney　　　　　(　　)
   2) nephron　　　　(　　)
   3) urine　　　　　(　　)
   4) ureter　　　　　(　　)
   5) urinary bladder　(　　)
   a. one of the two tubes which take the urine from the kidneys and to the urinary bladder
   b. a typically yellowish fluid stored in the bladder and secreted through urethra

The Urinary System

    c. each of the functional unit in the kidney, consisting of glomerulus, Bowman's capsule and associate tubules
    d. a sac where urine collects from the kidneys and through the ureter before discharging out of the body
    e. either of the two bean shaped organs situated on either side of the spine behind the abdomen that remove waste products into the urine

5. Select Japanese for each word.
    1) kidney   (　　)
    2) nephron   (　　)
    3) urine   (　　)
    4) ureter   (　　)
    5) urethra   (　　)
    a. 尿   b. 尿道   c. 腎臓
    d. 腎単位   e. 尿管

Nephron —ネフロン（腎単位）

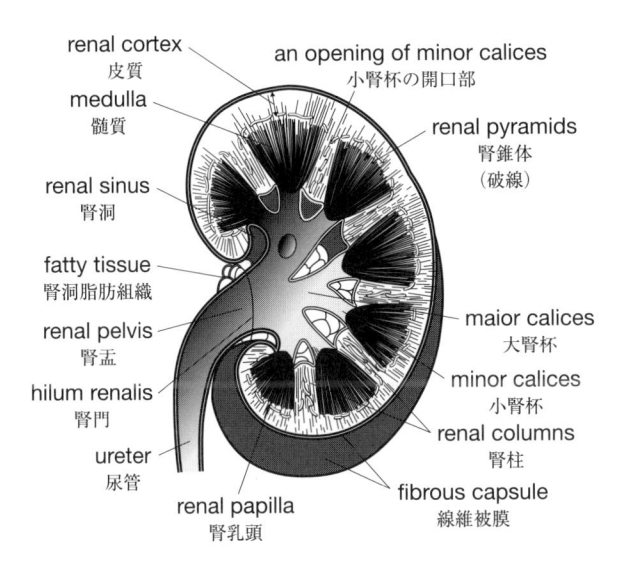

Diagram labels:
- renal cortex 皮質
- medulla 髄質
- renal sinus 腎洞
- fatty tissue 腎洞脂肪組織
- renal pelvis 腎盂
- hilum renalis 腎門
- ureter 尿管
- renal papilla 腎乳頭
- an opening of minor calices 小腎杯の開口部
- renal pyramids 腎錐体（破線）
- maior calices 大腎杯
- minor calices 小腎杯
- renal columns 腎柱
- fibrous capsule 線維被膜

The structure of nephrons makes them able to carry on their function of urine formation. Because the walls of the glomerular capillaries and of Bowman's capsules are very thin membranes, water and dissolved substances (except albumin and other blood proteins) filter rapidly out of the blood in the glomeruli into Bowman's capsules. This filtrate then trickles down the convoluted tubules; and as it does so, a large part of the water goes back into the blood, that is, is reabsorbed into capillaries around the tubules. Dissolved substances (solutes) also leave the tubule filtrate to return to the blood. Glucose, for instance, is entirely reabsorbed, so that none of it is wasted by being lost in the urine.

糸球体毛細血管

濾過液

溶質

The Urinary System

Like glucose, sodium chloride and other salts filter out of glomerular blood. Unlike glucose, however, salts are only partially reabsorbed from the tubule filtrate. The amount reabsorbed varies from time to time. When, for example, you salt food heavily, your kidneys reabsorb less salt than when you use salt sparingly. Thus, your body gets rid of excess salt by way of the urine, and in this way tends to keep the blood's salt concentration normal. This is an extremely important matter because cells are damaged by either too much or too little salt in the fluids around them.

塩化ナトリウム

加塩する

再吸収する

To summarize, we can say that three processes in succession accomplish the task of urine formation:

連続して

1. *Filtration*—of water and dissolved substances out of the blood in the glomeruli into Bowman's capsules

溶解物質

2. *Reabsorption*—of water and dissolved substances out of the kidney tubules back into the blood (Note that this process prevents substances needed by the body from being lost in the urine. Usually 97% to 99% of the water filtered out of the glomerular blood is retrieved from the tubules.)

3. *Secretion*—of hydrogen ions (H^+), potassium ions (K^+), and certain drugs (for example, penicillin)

水素イオン, カリウムイオン
ペニシリン

Let's pronounce medical English terms.

1. filtration   2. reabsorption   3. secretion
4. glomerulus

Review questions

1. What structure do the walls of the glomerular and of Bowman's capsules

Nephron

    have and how useful is that structure?
2. What elements of urine are filtrated in the tubule?
3. What are three processes in urine formation?
4. Fill the appropriate word in the blanks.

    The structure of nephrons makes them able to carry on their function of urine formation. Because the walls of the glomerular capillaries and of (   ) are very thin membranes, water and dissolved substances filter rapidly out of the blood in the (   ) into Bowman's capsules. This filtrate then trickles down the convoluted (   ) ; and as it does so, a large part of the water goes back into the (   ), that is, is reabsorbed into capillaries around the tubules. Dissolved substances (solutes) also leave the tubule filtrate to return to the blood. Glucose, for instance, is entirely reabsorbed, so that none of it is wasted by being lost in the (   ).

The Urinary System

医学英語の常識（8）
略語，略語，略語

　ハムレットのセリフ"Word, word, word."（ことば，ことば，ことば）をもじっていえば，医学領域では，"Abbreviation, abbreviation, abbreviation."（略語，略語，略語）といえるだろうか．

　たとえば，エイズという略語は学校教育でも，規模の小さい医院に貼られた感染防止のためのポスターまで日本中を席捲して久しい．エイズは，acquired immunodeficiency syndrome（後天性免疫不全症候群）の省略語 AIDS を音読みしたものである．この症候群を引き起こすウイルスは，1983年フランスで LAV（lymphadenopathy-associated virus）として，1984年アメリカで HTLV-III（the human T-lymphotrophic virus type III）として別に発見された．このウイルスは，RNA（ribonucleic acid：リボ核酸）を遺伝子としてもち，逆転写酵素によって DNA（deoxyribonucleic acid）を合成し，T-helper cell（tranfer cell：転移細胞）に特異的に感染し，人の免疫機構を破壊してしまう．その結果，感染者は通常は重大な事態とはならない菌にも感染しやすくなり（opportunistic infection：日和見感染），死に至るのである．syndrome はギリシア語に由来し，ともに（syn-）+ 走る（drome）という意味である．それは同一の原因，同一の症状，経過をたどる"病気（disease）"とは違って，外の器官にも同時に一連の症状・病的状態の徴候を示すことから，その治療も容易ではない[1]．

　私たちの周辺には医療関連の略語が散見される．たとえば，AED, ICU, ER, CT, ADL, SARS, BSE, 最近では iPS 細胞[2] などなど，一般の人にもよく知られた略語がある．とくに，日進月歩の医学，戦場のような医療の場では簡潔な略語が頻用されるのはもっともである．しかし，以下の事柄を知って略語を使用する必要があるだろう．

① 各職場に特有の略語，日本でのみ共通する略語，世界的に承認されている略語があるので，むやみに乱用しないこと．
② ひとつの略語に，別の意味をもつ複数の用語があること．たとえば，ある医学英語辞書では，上記 ER には 23 の英語が表記されている．
③ 医学英語の学習において初歩の段階では，フルスペリングを知る努力が必

要である.

注
1) Appendixには，比較的基本的な略語を選び，その代表的なフルスペリングを掲載した．
2) Appendix参照．

CHAPTER 9
The Nervous System　神経系

Constitution of the nervous system　神経系の構成

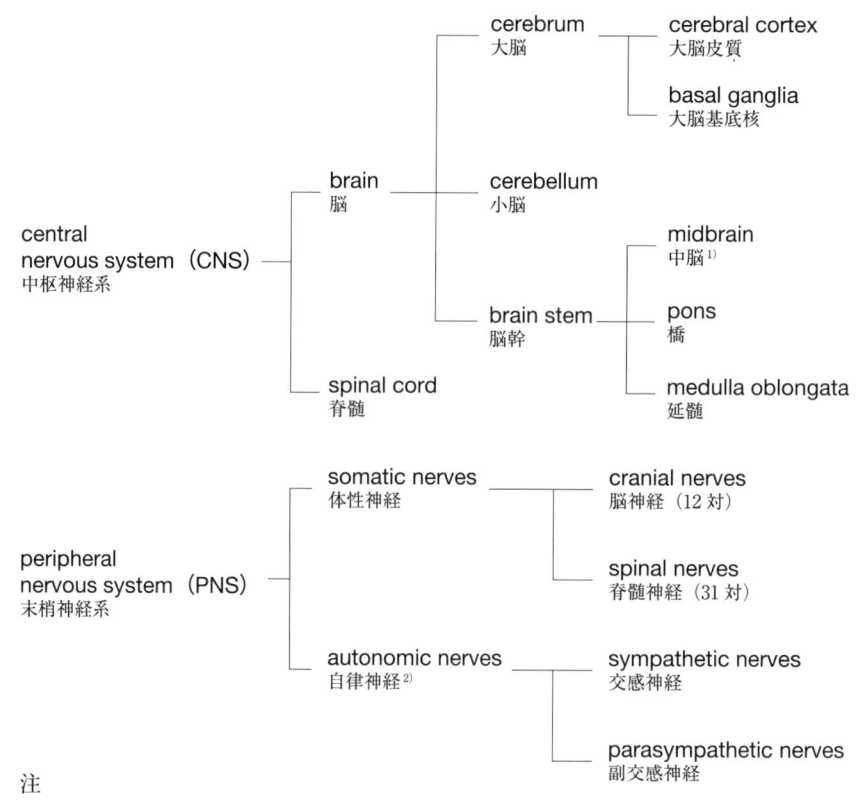

- central nervous system (CNS) 中枢神経系
  - brain 脳
    - cerebrum 大脳
      - cerebral cortex 大脳皮質
      - basal ganglia 大脳基底核
    - cerebellum 小脳
    - brain stem 脳幹
      - midbrain 中脳 [1]
      - pons 橋
      - medulla oblongata 延髄
  - spinal cord 脊髄

- peripheral nervous system (PNS) 末梢神経系
  - somatic nerves 体性神経
    - cranial nerves 脳神経（12 対）
    - spinal nerves 脊髄神経（31 対）
  - autonomic nerves 自律神経 [2]
    - sympathetic nerves 交感神経
    - parasympathetic nerves 副交感神経

注
1) midbrain = mesencephalon
2) autonomic nervous system ともいう．PNS の解剖学的分類は脳神経と脊髄神経に，機能的には体性神経と自律神経に分類される．

Background Information

The nervous system functions to enable the body to respond to stimuli from the environment and to perform life functions.　The functional unit of the nervous system is the nerve cell, the neuron.

刺激．単数形：stimulus

神経，ニューロン

The neuron consists of a cell body which contains the nucleus and has numerous tree-like extensions called dendrites.　These functions to receive and conduct impulses toward the cell.　A long fiber called the axon serves to conduct of relay the nerve impulses away from the cell body.　What is frequently called a nerve is in fact a bundle of axons.　Stimuli are received by structures called receptors.

核

樹状突起

軸索

レセプタ/受容器

Receptors may be specialized for reception of pressure, heat, cold, or other stimuli.　Electrical and chemical changes in the neuron transmit the impulse from the dendrite to the axon.　The gap from the nerve endings of the axon to the dendrites of the next neuron is known as synapse.　The impulse is able to bridge this gap and pass from neuron to neuron until it terminates in a structure capable of reacting to the stimuli.　These are known as effectors.　When this pathway to the impulse includes passages through a nerve center, it is known as reflex arc.

シナプス

効果器

反射弓

One division of the nervous system is the central nervous system which consists of the brain and spinal cord.　The cerebrum of the brain controls the higher processes and senses; the cerebellum controls the voluntary reflexes.

中枢神経系
[spáinl kɔ́:rd]

The other division of the nervous system, peripheral, consist of the cranial nerve and spinal cord and

[pərifərəl]

[créiniəl]

The Nervous System

the autonomic nervous structure. This latter structure serves the internal organs and controls such activities as digestion, circulation, respiration, excretion, reproduction, and the endocrine gland activity.

排泄
生殖,内分泌腺
［出 典 A, p.ii: R47 ～ p.iii: L30］

Let's pronounce medical English terms.

1. peripheral nervous system
2. autonomic nervous system（アクセント注意）
3. neuron   4. dendrite

Review questions

1. Explain the main function of the central nervous system briefly.
2. Explain the main sections of the autonomic nervous system briefly.
3. Select the appropriate word to be filled in the blanks.
   1) The central nervous system consists of the (　　) and the (　　).
   2) The (　　) consist of the cranial nerves and the spinal nerves.
   3) Receptors are able to respond to heat, cold or other external (　　) and makes the (　　) react in a particular way.

   a. the central nervous system
   b. the peripheral nervous system
   c. the autonomic nervous system
   d. sympathetic nervous system
   e. body   f. brain   g. cerebellum
   h. spinal cord   i. stimuli   j. effectors

4. Write the complete spelling of CNS and PNS.
   1) CNS (　　　　　　　　　　　　　　　　)
   2) PNS (　　　　　　　　　　　　　　　　)
5. Fill in the blanks in the figure with an appropriate word.

Background Information

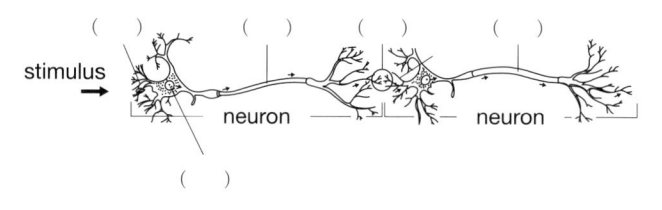

```
(   )        (   )        (   )        (   )
stimulus →  [neuron]              [neuron]
                 (   )
```

a. axon   b. dendrite   c. synapse   d. nucleus

The Nervous System

Spinal cord — 脊髄

The spinal cord occupies a protected location inside the spinal column. Nervous tissue is not a sturdy tissue. Even moderate pressure can kill nerve cells, so nature safeguards the chief organs made of this tissue — the spinal cord and the brain — by surrounding them with a tough, fluid-containing membrane (the meninges), and then by surrounding the membrane with bones. The *spinal meninges* form a tube-like covering around the spinal cord and line the vertebrae......

丈夫な組織

髄膜（単数形：meninx）

They are the dura mater (lines the vertebrae), the pia mater (covers the cord), and the arachnoid membrane between them. This middle layer of the meninges, the arachnoid membrane, resembles a cobweb with fluid filling in its spaces. (The word arachnoid means cobweblike. It comes from Arachne the name of the girl who was changed into a spider because she boasted of the fineness of her weaving. At least, so an ancient Greek myth tells us.)

硬膜
軟膜，くも膜

くもの巣，アラクネ

ギリシア神話

If you are of average height, your spinal cord is about 17 or 18 inches long. It lies inside the spinal column in the spinal cavity and reaches from the occipital bone down to the bottom of the first lumbar vertebra. (Place your hands on your hips and they will line up with your fourth lumbar vertebra; your spinal cord ends shortly above this level). The spinal meninges, however, continue down almost to the end of the spinal column — an important fact for a physician to know, because it means that he can do a lumbar puncture without fear of damaging the cord.

後頭骨

医師（内科医）
腰椎穿刺

注）脊椎腔の髄膜三層にはそれぞれ次のように意味がある．
dura（hard：厳しい）+ mater（mother：母親）= 厳しい母
pia（render：優しい）+ mater = 優しい母
arachnoid + mater（membrane）= arachn-：蜘蛛 + oid：〜のような = 蜘蛛の巣の母

Let's pronounce medical English terms.

1. spinal cord   2. meninges   3. dura mater
4. pia mater   5. arachnoid membrane

Review questions

1. How is the spinal cord guarded?
2. How long is your spinal cord, if you are of average height?
3. Does the spinal meninges go down to the end of the column?
4. Write an appropriate word in the blanks.
   a. arachnoid membrane   b. dura mater
   c. pia mater   d. skull

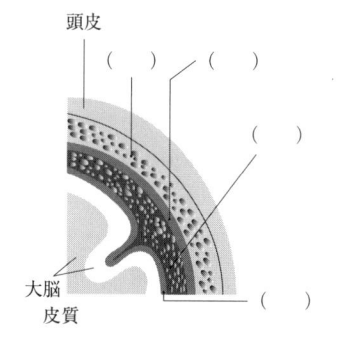

5. From what comes the word, arachnoid membrane?

The Nervous System

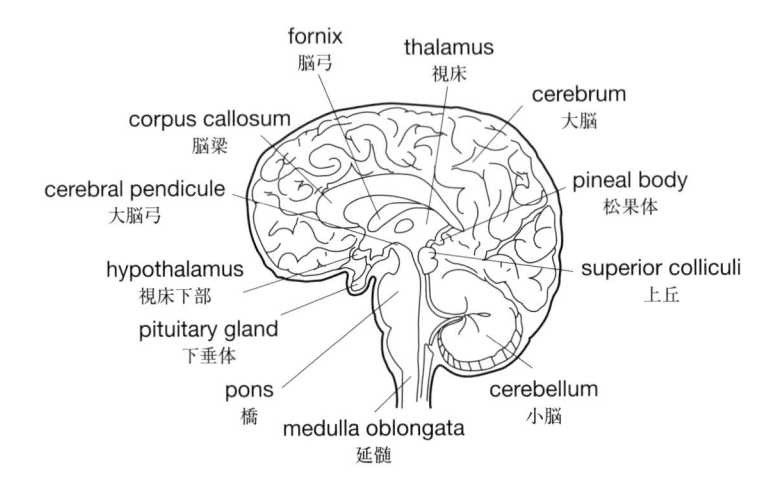

Brain —脳

```
           fornix    thalamus
           脳弓      視床
                              cerebrum
corpus callosum               大脳
脳梁
                              pineal body
cerebral pendicule            松果体
大脳弓
                              superior colliculi
hypothalamus                  上丘
視床下部
pituitary gland
下垂体
       pons              cerebellum
       橋                小脳
           medulla oblongata
           延髄
```

Background Information

Brain is the master control center of the body. The brain constantly receives information from the senses about conditions both inside the body and outside it. The brain rapidly analyzes this information 感覚 and then sends out messages that control body func- 情報分析する tions and actions. This brain also stores information from past experience, which makes learning and remembering possible. In addition, the brain is the source of thoughts, moods, and emotions.

The human brain is a grayish-pink, jellylike ball with many ridges and grooves on its surface. A new- 陵, 溝 born baby's brain weighs less than 0.5 kilogram. By the time a person is 6 years old, the brain has reached its full weight of about 1.4 kilograms. Most of the brain cells are present at birth, and so the increase in weight comes mainly from growth of the cells. During this six-year period, a person learns and acquires new behavior patterns at the fastest rate in life.

A network of blood vessels supplies the brain with the vast quantities of oxygen and food that it requires. The human brain makes up only about 2 per cent of the total body weight, but it uses about 20 per cent of the oxygen used by the entire body when at rest. The brain can go without oxygen for only three to five minutes before serious damage results.

The brain is located at the upper end of the spinal cord. This cable of nerve cells extends from the neck about two-thirds the way down the backbone. The spinal cord carries messages between the brain and other parts of the body. In addition, 12 pairs of nerves connect the brain directly with certain parts of the body.

The brain works somewhat like both a computer and a chemical factory. Brain cells produce electrical signals and send them from cell to cell along pathways called *circuits*. As in a computer, these electrical circuits receive, process, store, and retrieve information. Unlike a computer, however, the brain creates its electrical signals by chemical means. The proper functioning of the brain depends on many complicated chemical substances produced by brain cells.

The brain has three main divisions: (1)the cerebrum, (2)the cerebellum, and (3)the brain stem. Each part consists chiefly of nerve cells, called *neurons*, and supporting cells, called *glia*.

The Nervous System

The function of the brain —脳の働き
The followings are the main functions of the brain.
1. receiving sensory messages
2. controlling movements
3. the use of language
4. producing emotions
5. thinking and remembering
6. regulating body processes

The function of the brain in the use of language
言語の使用における脳の働き

Many parts of the brain are involved in our use of language. The centers of vision and hearing enable us to understand written or spoken words. The motor cortex and the cerebellum order the proper movements of the lips, tongue, and other organs of speech. In addition, two areas of the association cortex are vital in the use of language. They are *Wernicke area* in the temporal lobe and *Broca area* in the frontal lobe. Scientists estimate that about 97 per cent of all people have these two areas only in the left cerebral hemisphere. The remaining 3 per cent have the language areas in both hemispheres.

When we hear a word, Wernicke area interprets the meaning of the sound pattern. When we read a word, a brain area called the *angular gyrus* converts the visual image into its associated sound, which Wernicke area then interprets. Wernicke area also formulates the sentences we speak. Broca area supplies detailed instructions for the muscle movements required for speaking a particular word. These instruc-

運動皮質

ウェルニッケ（独：神経科医，1848～1906）
ブローカ（仏：解剖学者，外科医，1824～1880）
左大脳半球

角回

The work of the brain: in the use of language

tions are sent to the motor cortex, which orders the movements.

［出典 B, Vol.2, p.565: R21 ～ p.566: L4 （一部抜粋）］

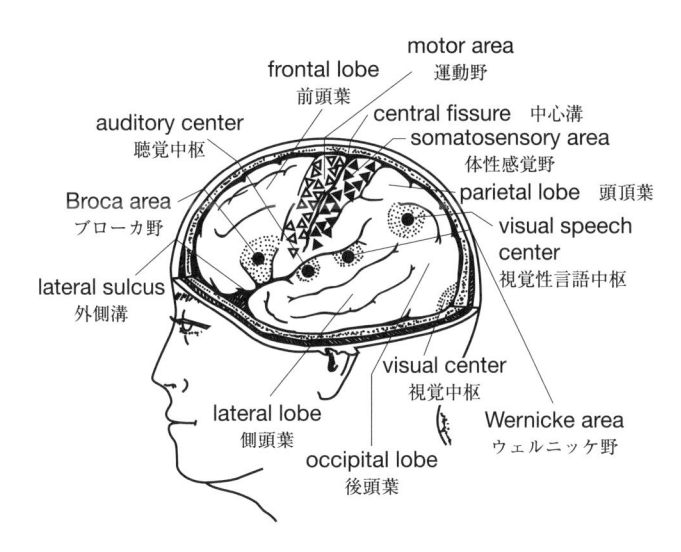

- motor area 運動野
- frontal lobe 前頭葉
- central fissure 中心溝
- somatosensory area 体性感覚野
- auditory center 聴覚中枢
- parietal lobe 頭頂葉
- Broca area ブローカ野
- visual speech center 視覚性言語中枢
- lateral sulcus 外側溝
- visual center 視覚中枢
- lateral lobe 側頭葉
- Wernicke area ウェルニッケ野
- occipital lobe 後頭葉

The Nervous System

Let's pronounce medical English terms

1. cerebrum
2. glia
3. cerebellum（アクセント注意）
4. Wernicke area
5. Broca area
6. angular gyrus

Review questions

Fill the blanks with the appropriate parts in English.

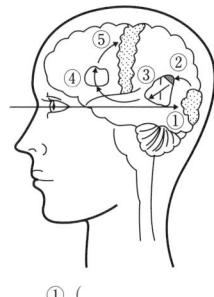

① (   )
② (   )
③ (   )
④ (   )
⑤ (   )
⑥ (   )

Brain death and Organ transplantation　脳死と臓器移植
(1) Histrory　臓器移植の歴史

　Organ transplantation is the moving of an organ from one body to another, or from a donor site on the patient's own body, for the purpose of replacing the recipient's damaged or absent organ.　The emerging field of regenerative medicine is allowing scientists and engineers to create organs to be re-grown from the patient's own cells (stem cells, or cells extracted from the failing organs.)　Organs and/or tissues that are transplanted within the same person's body are called autografts[1].　...　Organs that can be transplanted are the heart, kidneys, liver, lungs, pancreas, intestine, and thymus.　Tissues include bones, tendons (both referred to as musculoskeletal grafts), cornea, skin, heart valves, and veins.　Worldwide, the kidneys are the most commonly transplanted organs, while musculoskeleletal transplants outnumber them by more than tenfold.

　The heart was a major prize for transplant surgeon. But, as well as rejection issues the heart deteriorates within minutes of death, so any operation would have to be performed at great speed.　The development of the heart-lung machine was also needed.　Lung pioneer James Hardy attempted human transplantation in 1964, but as a premature failure of the recipient's heart caught Hardy with no human donor, he used a chimpanzee heart, which failed very quickly.

　The first success was achieved December 3, 1967 by Christian Barnard in Cape Town, South Africa.　Louis Washkansky, the recipient, survived for eighteen days

提供者

臓器受容者

再生医療

幹細胞
欠陥臓器

自家移植片 =
autogenic graft

〔出典 F〕
外科医

心肺装置

〔tʃimpænziː〕

外科医（1922-2001）

The Nervous System

amid what many saw as a distasteful publicity circus. The media interest prompted a spate of heart transplants. Over a hundred were performed in 1968-69, but almost all the patients died within sixty days. Barnard's second patient, Philip Blaiberg, lived for 19 months.

As the rising success rate of transplans and modern immunosuppression make transplants more common, the need for more organs has become critical. Advances in living-related donor transplants have made that increasingly common. Additionally, there is substantive research into xenotransplantation or transgenic organs; although these forms of transplant are not yet being used in humans, clinical trials involving the use of specific cell types have been conducted with promising results, such as using porcine islets of Langerhans to treat type one diabetes. However, there are still many problems that would need to be solved before they would be feasible options in patients requiring transplants.

Recently, researchers have been looking into means of reducing the general burden of immunosuppression. ... and in general, reduced immunosuppression increases the risk of rejection and decreases the risk of infection.

不快感を覚える評判の曲芸として見ていた最中に（比喩表現）

免疫抑制薬
非常に不可欠な
生きて適応できるドナーの移植
異種移植（注参照）
遺伝子導入の器官（他から特定のDNAを胚細胞の卵核内に人工的に導入された）
〔áɪlət〕
〔láːŋərháːns〕
適した選択

注）移植には，自家移植片のほか，自己以外の組織を移植する他家移植片（allograft）つまり，
　・同種片（allogenic graft）：人間の組織
　・異種片（xenogenic）：人間以外の組織
　・同系移植片（syngenic graft）：卵生双生児，近交系動物組織

・人工移植片（artificial graft）：形成術，人工的な素材がある．

(2) Organ transplantation in Japan　日本における臓器移植

The "Organ Transplantation Law" took effect on October 16, 1997 and legalized transplanting organs from brain dead donors in Japan. Approximately 30 years after the world's first heart transplant in South Africa, and over a decade after the establishment of United Network Organ Sharing (UNOS), "organ transplanting from brain dead donors" was finally made possible-something that had already been recognized as normal procedure in other advanced countries. It has been said that organ transplanting would not come to fruition in Japan because of the unique view of the Japanese people toward life, death, ethics, and religion. Ever since the Wada heart transplant in 1968, there has been a deep-rooted sense of apprehension toward brain death and transplanting. Now, as light flickers at the end of the tunnel, it is time to reconsider the issues facing organ transplantation in Japan and to discuss the steps that need to be taken.

臓器移植法
効力を発する
脳死提供者

全米臓器分配ネットワーク

成果があがる，実を結ぶ
倫理
宗教

トンネルの出口で（比喩表現）

注）2010年7月17日の改正移植・臓器法施行後，脳死臓器提供に必須であった「本人の書面による意思表示」がなくても，「提供しない」という意思表示がなければ，家族の承諾のみで提供できるようになった．また，15歳未満の子供からの脳死臓器提供も可能となった．改正法通過後の脳死臓器提供は，以前より確実に増加している．

(3) Views on Brain Death　脳死に関する見解

According to the World Health Organization (WHO), only a few countries such as Pakistan and Ro-　〔pǽkɪstæ̀n〕

111

The Nervous System

mania do not recognize brain death as human death. In Japan, while the Organ Transplantation Law has been enacted, brain death is acknowledged as human death only when a transplant is to be performed.

 Brain death refers to a condition in which the function of the entire brain, including the brain stem that controls respiration, is irreversibly lost due to occurrences such as head trauma and cerebral apoplexy. The advent of respirators made it possible to temporarily maintain the heart beat even after the loss of cerebral function, but the heart will eventually stop beating in a few days.

 The vegetative state is the condition in which all or some of the cerebral functions are lost and the patient loses consciousness. However, the functions of the brain stem remain, spontaneous respiration is possible in many cases, and sometimes recovery occurs. Therefore a vegetative state is fundamentally different from brain death. Brain death will only be declared if organic injury is observed in the brain with attributable cause and if the following are met:

1. Deep coma
2. Dilated an fixed pupils
3. Loss of brain stem activity
4. Flat brain waves
5. Loss of spontaneous respiration
6. Two or more doctors with requisite expertise and experience confirm no changes after a second test conducted six or more hours later.

 Brain death cannot be declared in persons with drug intoxication, low body temperature, or endo-

Margin notes: 〔ruméinia〕 制定される 脳卒中 出現 拍動 植物状態 帰することのできる原因 薬物中毒

crine/metabolic diseases.

This evaluation is considered to be medically certain. However, when respiration and blood flow are still present or when spinal reflexes cause movement in the limbs, brain death may be difficult to evaluate for Japanese who have recognized heart arrest (confirmation of the three signs: 1. Cessation of heart beat; 2. Cessation of spontaneous respiration; and 3. Loss of light reflex/dilated pupils) as human death.

心停止
中断
拡張瞳孔の対光反射
〔出典 G〕

To make sure of your reading.
1. What is the purpose of organ transplantation?
2. Who succeeded the organ transplant in the world and when?
3. What made the need of more organs very important?
4. What kind of transplantation is Xenotransplantation?
5. When was in force Organ Transplantation Law in Japan?
6. Why did not the organ transplantation bear to fruit in Japan?
7. List up the standards of the brain death.

The Nervous System

医学英語のルーツ—ギリシア神話（6）
蜘蛛とクモ膜とアラクネ

　脊髄と脳髄を取り巻く三層の中間の膜の由来は，英文中にギリシア神話に登場する織物の巧みな少女，アラクネ（Arachne）に因むと説明されている．では，なぜ少女は蜘蛛に変えられてしまったのだろう？

　神話によると，アラクネはこともあろうにあの知恵と学問と技芸と戦いの女神アテナと機織りの競争をしたそうな．彼女の母親は早世したが，父親は，機織りの好きな娘に貴重な液で染めた高価な糸を惜しまず与えては可愛がった．少女は毎日，機を織って暮らすうちに，'What one likes, one will do best.'（好きこそ物の上手なれ）で，その地方で並ぶものない機織りの名手となった．彼女は父親に可愛がられ，ただ織物だけに心を注いで過ごしていたためか，世間知らずの恐いもの知らず．「アテナ様と技比べをしても，決して負けはいたしませぬ」と公言した．とかく言葉は矢のように走るもの．ゼウスと肩を並べる実力者のアテナの耳に達した．

　カチンときた女神は老婆の姿に変えて足元をふらつかせながら少女のもとを訪れ，諭した．「お前は人間だし，若いだけが取り柄だ．自慢しないほうが身のためだよ」すると少女は言い放った．「ばあさんにとやかく言われたくないわ．どうしてもというなら女神をここへ連れてきて．受けて立つから」．怒り心頭に発したアテナはもちろん，即座に本当の姿を現した．

　技比べがはじまった．金糸，銀糸，高貴な紫色，微妙な淡い自然の色，ありとあらゆる色合いの糸を織り込み完成したふたりの織物に，人々は驚嘆した．アテナの織り模様は天地創造の様を，オリュンポスの十二神の鮮やかな艶やかな姿と，アテナイの町を巡る争いで，盾と槍を手に持ち，兜を被った雄雄しい（？）自らを描き，そしてオリーブの葉の冠が縁取られていた．それは奇跡にも似た見事さであった．一方，アラクネの織物は，神々の謀略，横暴のかぎりを精密に描き切っていた．たとえば，化け物のように変貌させられたあの美少女メドゥーサ（アテナの怒り故），白牛と化してフェニキア王の娘エウロペをさらっていくゼウス，偽の葡萄酒をエーリゴネに飲まして騙すバッカス（酒の神），人間の女ピュリュラーに半人半馬のケンタウロスを産ませているクロノス（ゼウスの父）などが織り込まれ，完璧な出来であった．

医学英語のルーツ―ギリシア神話 (6)

しかし,女神は女神である.威信にかけて負けを認めるわけにはいかない.アテナ神は(アドレナリン分泌過多で,aggressive な性格?),織物を切り裂き,アラクネの頭を打ちすえた.それでも,アラクネは女神に抵抗し(神への反逆罪に相当する?),逆に辱めに耐えられずとうとう首を括って死んでしまった.アテナの腹立ちはそれでも収まらない.「蜘蛛になって日がな一日,糸を紡いでいればいいのよ」とその死体にトリカブト(monkshood)の汁を撒いて,蜘蛛に変えてしまった,というわけ.

Arachne に因む医学英語

acotine (monkshood) poisoning トリカブト中毒:花の形が能楽の帽子の鳥兜に,英語は西洋の僧侶の帽子に似ていることから.
subarachnoid hemorrhage クモ膜下出血
arachnoid granulations クモ膜顆粒
subarchnoid cavity クモ膜下腔.接尾辞 -oid (= resemblance) は Appendix 参照.
subarachnoid block 脊椎麻酔.接尾辞 -oid は Appendix 参照.

CHAPTER 10
The Sense Organs　感覚器官

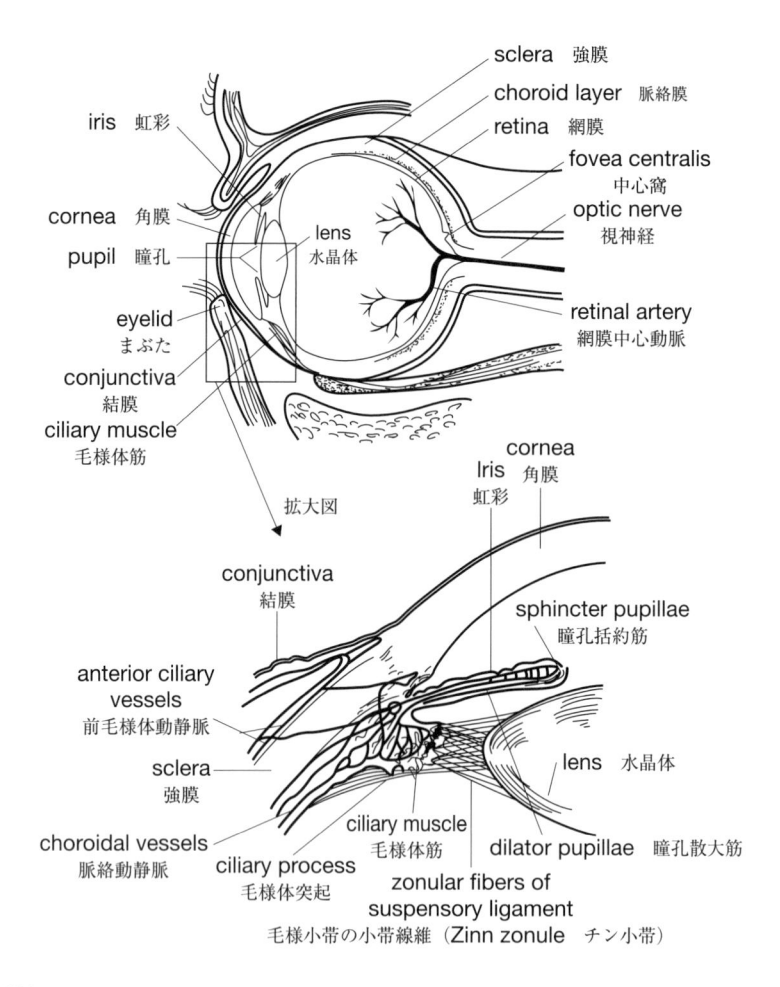

sclera　強膜
choroid layer　脈絡膜
retina　網膜
fovea centralis　中心窩
optic nerve　視神経
retinal artery　網膜中心動脈
iris　虹彩
cornea　角膜
pupil　瞳孔
lens　水晶体
eyelid　まぶた
conjunctiva　結膜
ciliary muscle　毛様体筋

拡大図

cornea　角膜
Iris　虹彩
conjunctiva　結膜
sphincter pupillae　瞳孔括約筋
anterior ciliary vessels　前毛様体動静脈
sclera　強膜
lens　水晶体
choroidal vessels　脈絡動静脈
ciliary muscle　毛様体筋
ciliary process　毛様体突起
dilator pupillae　瞳孔散大筋
zonular fibers of suspensory ligament
毛様小帯の小帯線維（Zinn zonule　チン小帯）

If you were asked to name the sense organs, what organs would you name? Can you think of any besides the eyes, ears, nose, and taste buds? Actually, ... receptors are generously scattered about in almost every part of the body. ... Stimulation of some receptors leads to the sensation of heat. Stimulation of other receptors gives the sensation of cold, and stimulation of still others gives the sensation of touch or pressure. When special receptors in the muscles and joints are stimulated, you sense the position of the different parts of the body and know whether they are moving or not and in which direction they are moving without even looking at them. Perhaps you have never realized that you have this sense of position and movement — a sense called *proprioception* or *kinesthesia*. 固有感觉，運動感觉
Let us turn our attention now to two complex and remarkable sense organs — the eyes and ears, and other sense organs, the nose, skin and tongue.

Eye — 目

The human eyeball measures only about 25 millimeters in diameter. Yet the eye can see objects as far away as a star and as tiny as a grain of sand. The eye can quickly adjust its focus between a distant point and a near one. It can be accurately directed toward an object even while the head is moving.

The eye does not actually see objects. Instead, it sees the light they reflect or give off. The eye can see in bright light and in dim light, but it cannot see in no light at all.

Light rays enter the eye through transparent tissues.

The Sense Organs

The eye changes the rays into electrical signals. The signals are then sent to the brain, which interprets them as visual images.

〔出典 B, Vol.6, p.468：L8 ～ L20〕

Focusing — 焦点調節

Light rays that enter the eye must come to a point on the retina for a clear visual image to form. However, the light rays that objects reflect or give off do not naturally move toward one another. Instead, they either spread out or travel almost parallel. The focusing parts of the eye — the cornea and the lens — bend the rays toward one another. The cornea provides most of the *refracting* (bending) power of the eye. After light rays pass through the cornea, they travel through the aqueous humor and the pupil to the lens. The lens bends the rays even closer together before they go through the vitreous humor and strike the retina. Light rays from objects at which the eyes are aimed come together at the *fovea centralis*, a tiny pit in the center of the macula. It is the area of sharpest vision. Light rays from objects to the sides strike other areas of the retina.

〔rétənə〕

屈折力

水様液〔éikwləs〕

硝子体液

〔sentréilis〕,〔mækjulə〕

The refracting power of the lens changes constantly as the eye shifts focus between nearby objects and distant ones. Light rays from nearby objects spread out, and those from distant objects travel nearly parallel. Therefore, the lens must provide greater bending power for the light rays from nearby objects to come together. This additional power is produced by a process called *accommodation*. In this process, one of the muscles of the ciliary body contracts, thereby re-

遠近調節

Focusing

laxing the fibers that connect the ciliary body to the lens.　As a result, the lens becomes rounder and thicker and thus more powerful.　When the eye looks at distant objects, the muscle of the ciliary body relaxes.　This action tightens the fibers that are connected to the lens, and the lens becomes flatter.　For this reason, the eye cannot form a sharp image of a nearby object and a distant one at the same time.

より平らになる

〔出典 B, Vol.6, p.470：R20 ～ p.471：L10〕

Let's pronounce medical English terms.

1. dendrite
2. kinesthesia
3. sclera
4. conjunctiva
5. vitreous humor
6. sphincter muscle

Review questions

1. What sense do we experience when your special receptors in the muscles and joint are stimulated?
2. How long is the human eyeball in diameter?
3. Does the eye actually see the objects?
4. If not, how can we see the objects?
5. What part of the eye has most of the bending power?
6. Why does the lens have great power for the light rays?

The Sense Organs

Ear — 耳

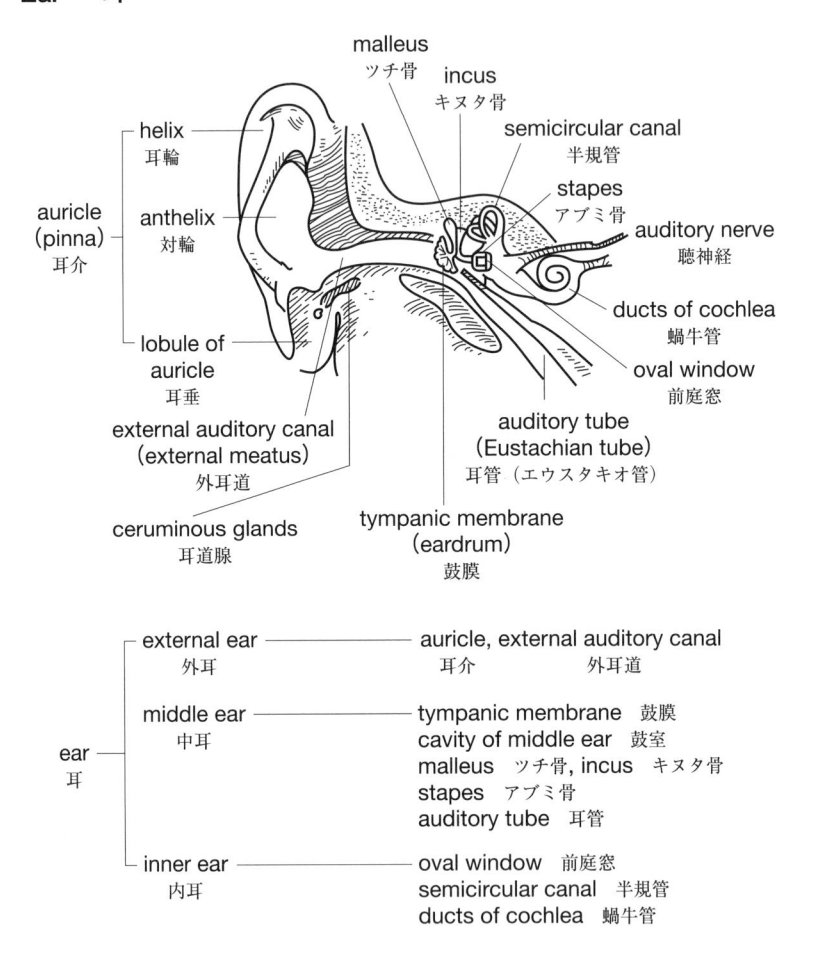

```
                    malleus
                    ツチ骨
                         incus
                         キヌタ骨
         helix                semicircular canal
         耳輪                  半規管
auricle  anthelix              stapes
(pinna)  対輪                   アブミ骨
耳介                                    auditory nerve
                                        聴神経
         lobule of                      ducts of cochlea
         auricle                        蝸牛管
         耳垂                            oval window
                                        前庭窓
         external auditory canal   auditory tube
         (external meatus)         (Eustachian tube)
         外耳道                     耳管（エウスタキオ管）
         ceruminous glands   tympanic membrane
         耳道腺                (eardrum)
                              鼓膜
```

	external ear 外耳	auricle, external auditory canal 耳介　外耳道
ear 耳	middle ear 中耳	tympanic membrane 鼓膜 cavity of middle ear 鼓室 malleus ツチ骨, incus キヌタ骨 stapes アブミ骨 auditory tube 耳管
	inner ear 内耳	oval window 前庭窓 semicircular canal 半規管 ducts of cochlea 蝸牛管

　The outer ear collects and funnels sound waves, （狭い所を）通す
which are air vibrations, through auditory canal to the 振動
eardrum.　The eardrum is a thin membrane (tissue)
stretched across the end of the auditory canal. When
sound waves strike the eardrum, it begins to vibrate.
The vibrations from the eardrum cause the three tiny

bones of the middle ear (hammer, anvil, and stirrup) to vibrate, too. malleus, incus, stapes の一般語

The vibration continues to the inner ear. Within the inner ear is the cochlea — a delicate organ shaped like a snail's shell filled with fluid and tiny nerve endings. When vibrations reach the cochlea, it sends nerve impulses to the auditory nerve leading to the brain. The brain interprets the various impulses as sound. Semicircular canals are also found in the inner ear. These are three tubes shaped like semicircles filled with fluid and nerve endings. Different body and head movements cause the fluid within the semicircular canals to move and change position, which in turn affects our sense of balance. The Eustachian tube connects the middle ear with the throat. The purpose of this tube is to permit equalization of air pressure in the middle ear. This is necessary so that the pressure on both sides of the eardrum will be the same.

蝸牛の殻

エウスタキオ管
〔juːsteiʃən〕

| Let's pronounce medical English terms. |

1. malleus 〔mǽliəs〕   2. incus 〔íŋkəs〕
3. stapes 〔stéɪpiz〕   4. ducts of cochlea
5. auditory ossicle

| Review questions |

1. What are the functions of the ear?
2. The following is the way of second conduction to the inner ear. Fill in the blanks with the name of the organs in Japanese.
   (a) external auditory canal 外耳道 → (b) eardurm (　　　) →
   (c) malleus ツチ骨 → (d) incus (　　　) → (e) stapes アブミ骨 →
   (f) oval window 前庭窓 → (g) ducts of cochlea (　　　)

The Sense Organs

Skin — 皮膚

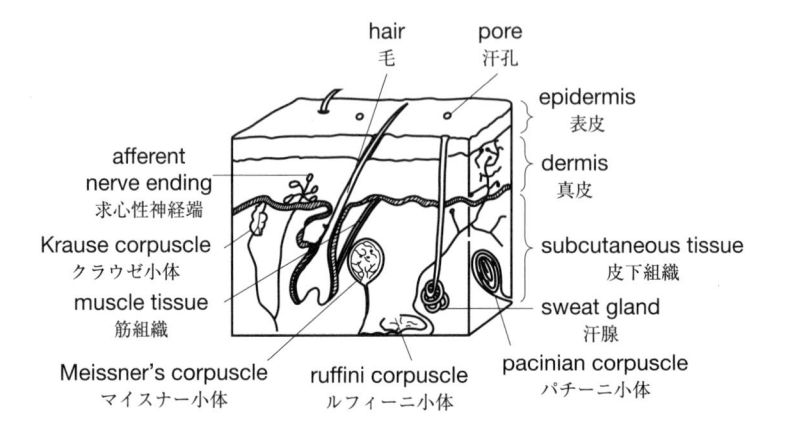

```
         hair    pore
          毛     汗孔
                      epidermis
                      表皮
                      dermis
afferent              真皮
nerve ending
求心性神経端
Krause corpuscle      subcutaneous tissue
クラウゼ小体            皮下組織
muscle tissue         sweat gland
筋組織                 汗腺
   Meissner's corpuscle   ruffini corpuscle   pacinian corpuscle
   マイスナー小体           ルフィーニ小体        パチーニ小体
```

    Skin is a soft outer covering of an animal, in particular a vertebrate. ... In mammals, the skin is the largest organ of the integumentary system made up of multiple layers of ectodermal tissue, and guards the underlying muscles, bones, ligaments and internal organs. Because it interfaces with the environment, skin plays a key role in protecting (the body) against pathogens and excessive water loss. Its other functions are insulation, temperature regulation, sensation, and the protection of vitamin D folates. Severely damaged skin will try to heal by forming scar tissue. This is often discoloured and depigmented.

哺乳動物
外皮（表皮）系
外胚葉組織

病原体
断熱化，体温調節

〔出典 H〕

Let's pronounce medical English terms.

1. epidermis   2. dermis   3. sweat gland
4. subcutaneous tissue

Nose ― 鼻

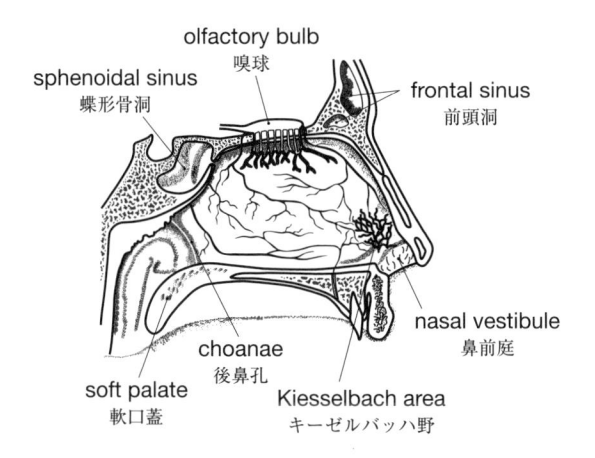

olfactory bulb
嗅球

sphenoidal sinus
蝶形骨洞

frontal sinus
前頭洞

nasal vestibule
鼻前庭

choanae
後鼻孔

soft palate
軟口蓋

Kiesselbach area
キーゼルバッハ野

The nose has an area of specialised cells which are responsible for smelling (part of the olfactory system). Another function of the nose is the conditioning of inhaled air, warming it and making it more humid. Hairs inside the nose prevent large particles from entering the lungs. Sneezing is usually caused by foreign particles irritating the nasal mucosa, but can more rarely be caused by sudden exposure to bright light (called the photic sneeze reflex) or touching the external auditory canal. Sneezing is a means of transmitting infections because it creates aerosols in which the droplets can harbour microbes.

嗅覚系

異物, 鼻粘膜

光性くしゃみ反射

エアロゾル（煙霧質）
小　　　　　滴
〔出典 I〕

Let's pronounce medical English terms.

1. sneeze　　2. nasal vestibule　　3. olfactory system
4. nasal mucosa

The Sense Organs

Tongue ― 舌

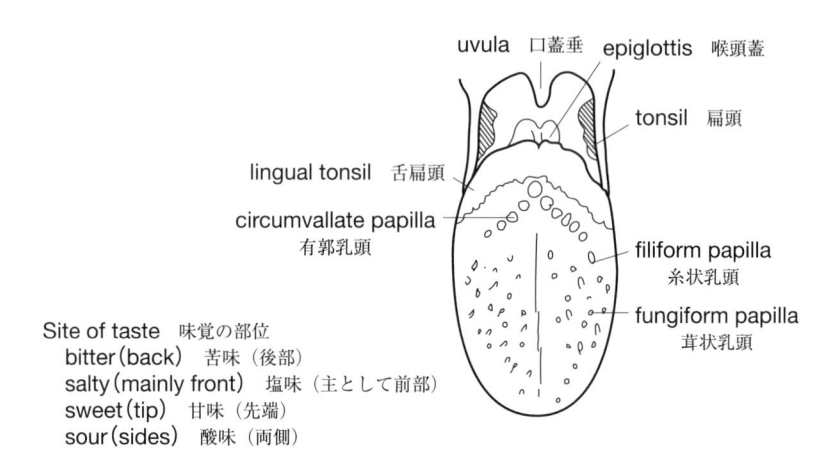

```
                            uvula 口蓋垂  epiglottis 喉頭蓋
                                          tonsil 扁桃
        lingual tonsil 舌扁桃
        circumvallate papilla
                   有郭乳頭
                                          filiform papilla
                                          糸状乳頭
                                          fungiform papilla
                                          茸状乳頭
   Site of taste   味覚の部位
      bitter (back)    苦味（後部）
      salty (mainly front)   塩味（主として前部）
      sweet (tip)    甘味（先端）
      sour (sides)   酸味（両側）
```

The tongue is a muscular hydrostat on the floors of the mouths of most vertebrates which manipulates food for mastication. It is the primary organ of taste, as much of the upper surface of the tongue is covered in papillae and taste buds. It is sensitive and kept moist by saliva, and is richly supplied with nerves and blood vessels. In humans a secondary function of the tongue is phonetic articulation. The tongue also serves as a natural means of cleaning one's teeth.	水床臓器 処理する 咀嚼する 乳頭 発話する 〔出典 J〕

| Let's pronounce medical English terms. |

1. lingual tonsil   2. papilla   3. phonetic articulation

The Doctor's Wife (華岡青洲の妻)

作者：有吉佐和子（1931-1984），作品出版年：1966
あらすじ： *The Doctor's wife* は，紀州上那賀郡名手荘にある貧乏医者の子青洲が，世界で初めて麻酔薬を開発し，紀州に並ぶ者のない名医として大成した過程を描いたものである．青洲は，文化2年10月，子宮癌の手術で全身麻酔に成功して以来，日本各地から外科医がはるばる青洲の門戸を叩くことになるほど栄達を極めた．作者，有吉佐和子は，名医が生まれる蔭で，麻酔薬通仙散の開発に競って身を献ずる姑於継と嫁加恵との確執をからませて，精緻な筆致で描いている．Readingは，実験体となった加恵が，その薬の副作用のために失明する場面である〔出典 K〕．

登場人物

Seisyu　花岡青洲（＝Umpei）
Kae　　加恵（青洲の妻）
Otsugi　於継（青洲の母）
Koriku　小陸（青洲の妹）

Early the next morning, the subject awake to a piercing pain in her eyes. ...　　さすような痛み
"Kae, what's wrong?"
"I'm sorry."
"Tell me how you feel.　Tell me everything."
"It's my eyes."
"What?"
"They hurt.　I have an awful pain in my head."...　　頭がずきずき痛む
　Otsugi left the room, found a towel, and went outside to the well where Koriku and several maids washing bunches of spring horseradishes.　　春ワサビダイコン（春

The Sense Organs

"Mother," called Koriku. "How is Kae?"

"She just got up."

"Really? That was quick."

"I'm sure everything that has happened to her also occurred in the last experiment with me. But she makes such a fuss."

"Why? What is it?"

"She's complaining that her eyes hurt. I suppose a cold compress will help."

"Do you mean for her eyes?" Koriku's face became contorted with fear.

"All those tears since Koben died have weakened them. That's what's the matter. Umpei is worried because he thinks it's been caused by his medicine. Why couldn't she keep quiet? Goodness, she's inconsiderate!"

"Mother!" exclaimed Koriku.

Startled by the loud accusing tone, Otsugi looked up and saw her gentle daughter transformed into an angry woman. The other women were also amazed.

"It's not on account of her tears! And it wasn't after Koben's death that her eyes became weak. Haven't you noticed, Mother? Kae's eyes were affected long before her child got sick. Do you think my patient forebearing sister-in-law would complain for nothing? Mother, you must tell Umpei immediately. If you don't, I will. Kae's eyes hurt because of the medicine she took two years ago."

Otsugi was stupefied, as if she had received the lash of a whip. And from her own daughter! As for this new revelation, she had truly not been aware of Kae's

大根の英訳）

大騒ぎをする

冷湿布

恐れでゆがむ

おとなしくしておく
思慮がない

とがめるような響きに

驚いて

しんぼう強い義姉（姉さん）

茫然となる
むちひとふり

problem. Suddenly, while her fingers were in the cold water, she began to shake in an uncontrollable fashion, which prevented her from stopping Koriku, who started for Seishu's room.

"If what Koriku said were true," she reasoned to herself, "... Why wasn't I affected by the drug? The experiment only proves how dull and insensitive I really am. An idiot. Now Kae will get all the glory for her sacrifice." She was feeling her age more than ever.

理由を考えた
実験
だるい
無感覚

Kae was given a sedative and a cold wet towel over a piece of silk to place on her eyes. Gradually, she stopped groaning. ... Toward noon the pain had definitely subsided enough for Kae to eat a bowl of porridge.

鎮静剤
紅絹裂（もみきれ）
かゆ

"Sorry you have to worry," she said to her husband.

"Do try to eat," he replied with much tenderness.

Kae sat up by herself and without being prodded began to compare the differences between the two experiments. Overall, she didn't feel too badly, although her head, arms, and legs still felt somewhat numb.

記憶を呼び起こすことなく

麻痺

"But......," she mumbled shyly, "around here......"

つぶやく

Through the covers she pointed to the area near her knee. "It hurts, as though I fell."

"I pinched you there. Very hard too. And you didn't budge."

つねる

They both laughed.

"Where's Mother?" she inquired after a time.

"She was tired so I told her to rest."

"I'm grateful to her. By the way ... which midnight is this?" In the bright daylight, Kae blinked several

目をまばたく

The Sense Organs

times through watery eyes but could not see her husband.

"Kae......" He gently helped her lie down again.

"Do they hurt?"

"Not as much."

"Are you sure?"

He lifted her eyelids to examine the pupils. There was no reaction. The thrill of success vanished. From his visibly downcast face, it was clear that the reality of the moment had reached him. The doctor had become a husband. Although Kae could not see it, the black mole on his throat was quivering, indicating that he was trying to fight back tears.

まぶた，瞳孔
反応

ほくろ
涙をおしもどす

Days passed. The pain diminished and the discharge of mucus ceased altogether. But Kae's sight was completely gone. In constant torment, Seishu's heart was now always with her, even when his mother died like a decayed leaf falling at last to the ground.

目やに，視力

朽ちた葉が落ちるように

To make sure of your reading.
1. Why Kae lost her eyesight?
2. When Otugi felt her age for the first time?
3. Why do you think Kae and Otsugi competed for the development of the anesthetic, Tusensan, for Seishu?

医学英語のルーツ―ギリシア神話（7）
心の目：知らずして父を殺し，母と結婚した息子，オイディプス

　感覚器官の目は，古来，文学作品や聖書で効果的な比喩表現として用いられてきた．たとえば，「目には目を……」（旧約聖書『出エジプト記』21 章 24 節）は目を奪われたならば，目だけを奪え，という過度の復讐の禁止を，「見ないで信ずるものは幸いである」（新約聖書『ヨハネによる福音書』20 章 29 節）は，実際に見えない存在を見る心の目への価値転換を示すように．

　ギリシア神話を題材としたソポクレスの悲劇『オイディプス王』[注]でも，目は劇的要素として重要な役割を果たしている．父王ライオスは最も権威あるデルポイの神託を受け，「もし子をもうければ，その子によって命を失うであろう」という運命にあった．そのため，子が生まれると「殺せ」と命じる．王妃イオカステは命だけは，と，家臣に山奥深くに捨てさせた．その子をコエイントス王の羊飼いが見つけて王宮に連れ帰ると，子に恵まれていない国の妃は喜んで自分の子供とする．その時，オイディプスの足が樹の幹につながれ膨れていたことから，オイディプス（Oidipus ＝ 英語 Oedipus: oidi- ＝ 膨れた＋ pus 足）と名付けられたのである．

　成長したオイディプスは，ある日友達からコリント王の本当の子供ではない，とからかわれ，妃に真相を尋ねる．否定しながらも悲しげな母の表情にもしや，とアポロン神の託宣を受ける．「故郷に帰るな．もし帰れば父を殺し，母と結婚するであろう」との神託であった．戻るに戻れず途方にくれて山中をさまよい歩くうちに細い三岐辻に出た．その時，数人の供を連れた老人に出くわし，互いに道を譲らず争いとなり，馬上の人が振り上げた刀を避けようとしてその人を殺してしまう．

　彼はそのままテーベの町に出るが，そのころテーベの町は恐慌に襲われていた．スフィンクスが人々に謎をかけ，答えられないと食い殺していたからだ．謎に答えた者には，この国の王を約束する，と書かれた辻板が立つ始末．彼は「朝 4 本足，昼 2 本足，夜 3 本足で歩く者は何者か？」と問われ「人間だ」と答えると，スフィンクスは自らを恥じて谷に身を投げて死んでしまった．

　町を救ったオイディプスは，約束によってテーベ王となる．そして母とは

知らずイオカステと結婚し，4人の子供をもうける．ところが今度は凶作が続き，悪疫が流行りはじめた．彼はデルポイの神託—先王ライオスを殺した者を国外へ追放せよ—のままに犯人を探す命令を出す．うすうす事実を悟ったイオカステは，オイディプスに「犯人を捕まえてもどうなることでしょう」と忠告をするが，常に彼は問題をあやふやにしておくことのできない性質であった．神話からはみ出すその人間性は現代に通じる人間であったといえよう．

かつての家来がよび出され，夫（息子）がすべてを知るその直前に，イオカステは自室に走り込み，腰のサッシュで首を括り死に果てる．追った彼は母を降ろし，その胸のブローチを外すや「目にしてはならぬ人を見，知りたいと願っていた人を見分けられなかったお前たち（＝目）は，もう誰の姿も見てはならぬ！」と，両眼の目をくりぬき，運命を呪って放浪の旅へテーベを出ていく．

このオイディプスの話から，フロイト（Sigmund Freud: 1856–1939）が「息子が母に対して無意識にいだく性的思慕」というエディプスコンプレックスを提唱し，人間の深層心理に光を当て，精神分析学の道を開いたことはよく知られた事実である．

注）オイディプスはギリシア語読み．エディプスは英語読み．「コロノスのオイディプス」（Oedipus at Colōnus）では，彼は許されてテーベの町へ戻る．

Oedipus に因む医学英語

Oedipus complex　幼児が異性の親に愛着し，同性の親に競争心や攻撃心をおぼえる．3〜4歳で生じ，6歳ころの潜伏期が始まると抑圧される．このコンプレックスがうまく解消されないと性格，性同一性のように，精神発達に影響を及ぼす．同じギリシア神話に因む Electra complex とよばれる場合もある．

Oedipas neurosis　エディプス神経症（エディプスコンプレックスが成年期まで続く）．

Oedipal period（phase）　エディプス期

Oedipism　エディピズム（エディプスコンプレックスが明らかに現れること）．

CHAPTER 11
Endocrine/Exocrine System
内分泌系，外分泌系

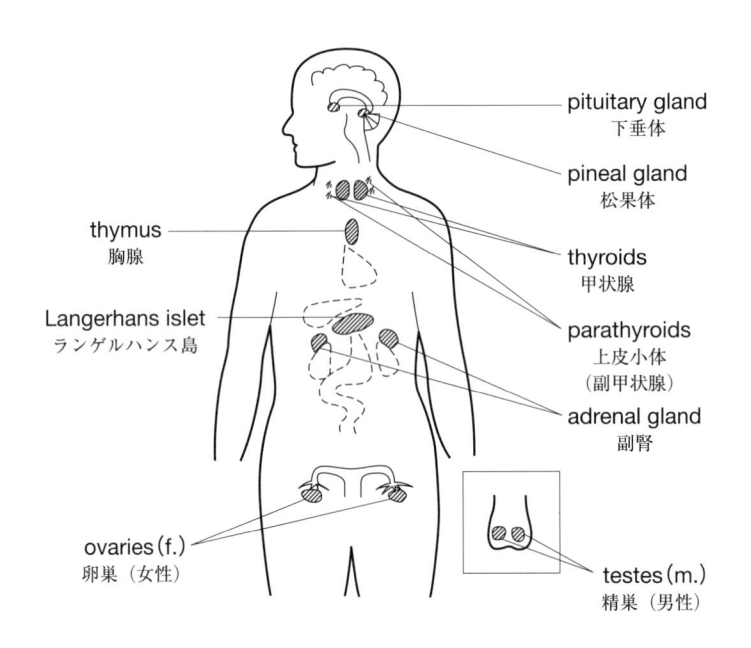

- pituitary gland 下垂体
- pineal gland 松果体
- thymus 胸腺
- thyroids 甲状腺
- Langerhans islet ランゲルハンス島
- parathyroids 上皮小体（副甲状腺）
- adrenal gland 副腎
- ovaries (f.) 卵巣（女性）
- testes (m.) 精巣（男性）

Endocrine glands — 内分泌腺

Endocrine glands, also called *ductless glands*, help the nervous system regulate various body activities. These glands produce and secrete chemical substances called *hormones*, which travel through the blood to all parts of the body. After a hormone arrives at its *target* — that is, the organ or tissue it affects — it causes certain actions to occur.

無道管腺

〔hɔ́:rmòun〕

標的

Hormones regulate such body processes as growth and development, and reproduction. Hormones also coordinate the body's responses to stress and help keep the chemical composition of the blood within normal range. In addition, hormones regulate the process by which the body changes food into energy and living tissue.

体作用

調整する
化学合成物

Most endocrine glands are organs and produce one or more hormones. Some of these glands consist of two or more parts, each of which secretes different hormones. Each of the two *adrenal glands*, for example, has two parts — the *cortex*, or outer layer, and the *medulla*, or inner layer. The cortex produces the hormones *cortisol* and *aldosterone*. The medulla secretes the hormones *epinephrine* and *norepinephrine*. Some endocrine glands are simply made up of tissue that forms part of another organ, such as the kidneys, pancreas, small intestine, and stomach.

副腎

コルチゾール, アルドステロン
エピネフリン, ノルエピネフリン
膵臓

The *pituitary gland* is one of the most important endocrine glands. It consists of two parts, the *anterior lobe* and the *posterior lobe*. The anterior lobe releases hormones that regulate the secretions of many other endocrine glands. For this reason, the pituitary is

下垂体 〔pət(j)ú:ətɛ́ri:〕
前葉
後葉

Endocrine/Exocrine System

sometimes called the *master gland*. The anterior lobe of the pituitary is controlled by a part of the brain known as the *hypothalamus*. The hypothalamus secretes *releasing hormones*, which cause the anterior lobe to discharge its hormones. The hypothalamus consists of nervous tissue. It forms the main link between the body's endocrine and nervous systems.

Some endocrine glands are not controlled by the pituitary or the nervous system. These glands, such as those that help maintain the normal chemical composition of the blood, respond to changes in the amounts of various chemicals. For example, the *parathyroid glands* secrete *parathormone* when the amount of calcium in the blood drops below the normal level. Parathormone causes a rise in the calcium level of the blood.

Diseases of the endocrine glands may cause them to secrete too much or too little of a hormone. Most cases of excess secretion result from tumors. Insufficient secretion occurs if a gland has been partly destroyed. This destruction may be caused by cancer, a decrease in the blood supply to the gland, or, in rare cases, infection. In many instances, the partial destruction of a gland results when the body's disease-fighting cells mistakenly attack healthy tissue.

支配力のある腺

視床下部

放出ホルモン

副甲状腺

副甲状腺ホルモン

腫瘍

〔出典 B, Vol.8, p.207：L69 ～ p.209：L21〕

| Let's pronounce medical English terms. |

1. hormone   2. medulla   3. pituitary gland
4. hypothalamus   5. parathyroid gland   6. parathormone

Review questions

1. What substances do endocrine glands secrete?
2. What happens, when the amount of a hormone changes?
3. What does 'endo-' mean?
4. Select the appropriate word to be filled in the blanks.
   1) The (   ) is one of the most important endocrine glands. It consists of two parts, the *anterior lobe* and the *posterior lobe*.
   2) The (   ) of the pituitary gland releases hormones that regulate the secretions of many other endocrine glands.
   3) The anterior lobe of the pituitary is controlled by a part of the brain known as the (   )
   4) The hypothalamus secretes (   ), which cause the anterior lobe to discharge its hormones.

   a. releasing hormone   b. medulla
   c. pituitary gland   d. hypothalamus
   e. parathyroid gland

Endocrine/Exocrine System

Exocrine glands — 外分泌腺

Exocrine glands, unlike endocrine glands, do not empty their secretions into the blood. Instead, their products are carried by ducts to the surface of the skin or other organs. The secretions perform various functions. The *sweat glands,* for example, secrete fluids that help cool the skin. The *sebaceous glands* supply oil that lubricates the skin. The *lacrimal glands* produce tears, which moisten the eyes. Other exocrine glands secrete substances that moisten and lubricate surfaces of organs within the body. Still others — glands that lie within the mouth, the stomach, and the intestine — help digest food.

生成物
汗腺
皮脂腺
すべすべさせる，涙腺

Certain exocrine glands secrete scents known as *pheromones,* which play an important role in communication among individuals in many animal species. The role in human behavior is more limited.

フェロモン〔férəmòun〕

Some exocrine glands consist of single cells. Others are made up of groups of tubes and *sacs* (baglike structures). Most exocrine glands release their secretions in response to stimulation of local nerve endings. But the secretions of some exocrine glands are controlled by hormones. For example, *gastrin,* a hormone secreted by the stomach, stimulates certain exocrine glands to release digestive juices. Exocrine glands, like endocrine glands, may be affected by various diseases that disrupt their secretions.

……に反応して

ガストリン（胃酸分泌を刺激するホルモン）

粉砕する

Glandlike structures — 腺様構造

The *thymus,* an organ in the chest, is often called a gland. This organ helps protect the body against dis-

胸腺

ease. Some scientists believe the thymus produces and releases one or more hormones, but researchers have not identified these secretions. Certain groups of *lymph nodes*, particularly those of the neck and armpit, are also called glands. But these structures do not produce secretions. Like the thymus, lymph nodes form part of the body's system of defense against disease.

リンパ節, 腋窩

| Let's pronounce medical English terms. |

1. sweat gland   2. sebaceous gland   3. thymus
4. lacrimal gland   5. pheromone

| Review questions |

1. How do most exocrine glands release their secretions?
2. Fill in the blanks with appropriate words below.
   1) The (　　) secrete fluids that help cool the skin.
   2) The (　　) produce tears, which moisten the eyes.
   3) (　　), a hormone secreted by the stomach, stimulates certain exocrine glands to release digestive juices.
   a. gastrin   b. lacrimal gland   c. sweat glands
   d. tears   e. the islet of Langerhans island

Endocrine/Exocrine System

Medical uses of hormones ― ホルモン療法

Physicians use hormones to treat people with *hormone deficiencies*. The body of a patient with such a condition cannot produce an adequate supply of one or more hormones. Hormone therapy enables a person to overcome many of the symptoms of various diseases. Such therapy cannot cure these diseases. It merely controls them. Hormone deficiency diseases include Addison's disease, diabetes mellitus, diabetes insipidus, and myxedema.

  ホルモン欠乏
  適切な供給
  ホルモン療法
  症状

  アジソン病，真性糖尿病，尿崩症
  粘液水腫

Certain other conditions which are not directly related to hormone deficiencies, may also be treated with hormones. These conditions include arthritis and asthma, for which many physicians prescribe cortisone.

  関節炎
  喘息，コルチゾンを処方する

In addition, hormones may be given to alter a function of the body in some way. Birth control pills, for example, contain synthetic female sex hormones. By taking these hormones, a woman alters the endocrine balance that controls the menstrual cycle. This alteration blocks *ovulation* (the release of eggs), thus making it almost impossible for pregnancy to occur.

  変える
  ピル（経口避妊薬）
  合成女性ホルモン

  排卵

Let's pronounce medical English terms.

1. hormone deficiency　2. diabetes mellitus　3. ovulation
4. pregnancy　5. synthetic female sex hormones

Review questions

1. What does the Greek word 'hormone' mean?
2. What function does medical use of hormone do?
3. Give some examples of the medical uses of hormones.

Medical uses of hormones

4. Select the appropriate Japanese.
    1) diabetes insipidus （　　）
    2) diabetes mellitus （　　）
    3) ovulation （　　）
    4) pregnancy （　　）
    5) symptom （　　）
    a. 排卵　　b. 妊娠　　c. 症状
    d. 尿崩症　e. 糖尿病

Endocrine/Exocrine System

医学英語の常識（9）
医学に貢献する fruit fly

　テキストも終わりに近づいてきた．いい古された諺を引用すると，本当に"Time flies like an arrow"（光陰矢の如し）である．皆さんは，そろそろ医学英語に馴染むようになったであろうか？

　さて，この諺をコンピュータで翻訳すると，「時バエは矢が好きである」「ハエの速度を矢のように計れ」「矢のようなハエの速度を計れ」というように訳されるからおもしろい．

　ところで，この諺をもじった次のような英文を見つけた．

　Fruit flies like a banana.

　訳してみよう．諺にならうと「果物はバナナのように飛ぶ」となる．

　しかし，正解は，「ショウジョウバエはバナナが好き」である．flies は'ハエ'という名詞の複数形であり，fruit fly は'ショウジョウバエ'という意味である．like は他動詞である．この文はショウジョウバエの好物がバナナであるところから，世に知られた諺をもじったものである．イギリスの某研究所の前に立てられた標示板に書かれているとか．

　では，"Time flies like an arrow."の動詞はなぜ三人称単数 flies なのか？ 主語が三人称の場合，動詞は s または es をつけた形になることを知っているだろう．では，その理由は？　ヒントにイギリス国家 '*God save the Queen*' を引用しよう．

　God save our gracious Queen,
　Long live our noble Queen,
　God save the Queen,
　Send her victorious,
　Happy and glorious,
　Long to reign over us,
　God save the Queen.

"God saves the Queen."ではないが，誤りではない．結論から先にいうと，"God save the Queen."は，"May God save the Queen."（神が女王陛下を助けられるように）という祈願文の省略形である．"God saves the Queen."（神が女王陛下を助けられる）という直接法による平叙文と，祈願文とを区別するために，英語では三人称の動詞にはsが残った，と考えることができるのだ．

　英語もその発達の初期の段階では，ドイツ語と同じように動詞も語尾変化をした．けれども長い時間の経過とともに英語はドイツ語と異なる変化をたどり，今は，三人称の動詞の現在形の語尾sに，その語尾変化の名残りをみることができる．

　ところで，このfruit flyの寿命は20日から80日近くであるが，その寿命はたった6個の遺伝子の組み合わせで決定されるという．fruit flyは短い寿命ながら立派に医学に貢献しているのだ．ちなみにネットで検索すると，fruit flyについてかなりの情報を得ることができるであろう．とくに遺伝学（genetics）ではfruit fliesがあたかも飛び回っているかのような活躍・貢献ぶりである．

CHAPTER 12
The Reproductive System　生殖系

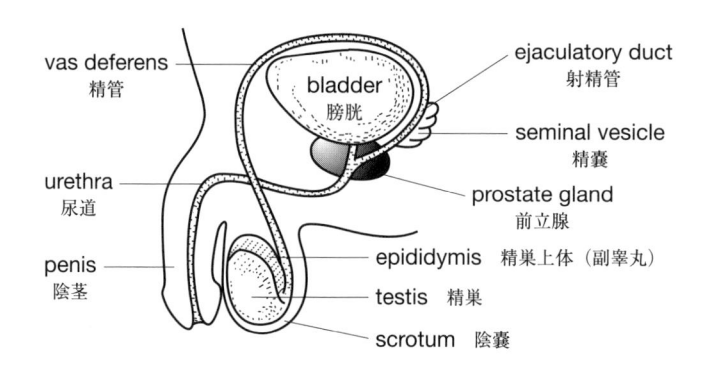

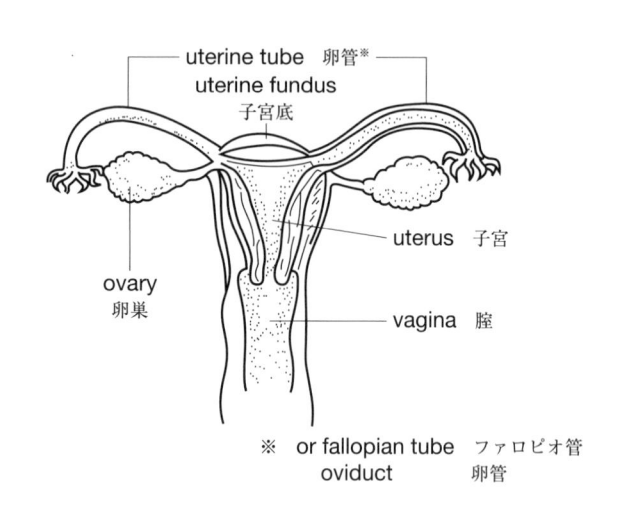

vas deferens　精管
bladder　膀胱
ejaculatory duct　射精管
seminal vesicle　精嚢
urethra　尿道
prostate gland　前立腺
penis　陰茎
epididymis　精巣上体（副睾丸）
testis　精巣
scrotum　陰嚢

uterine tube　卵管※
uterine fundus　子宮底
ovary　卵巣
uterus　子宮
vagina　腟

※　or fallopian tube　ファロピオ管
　　oviduct　卵管

Background Information

Fearfully and wonderfully made we truly are. Almost any one of the body's structures or functions might have inspired this statement, but of them all perhaps the reproductive systems best deserve such praise. Their achievement? The miracle of duplicating the human body. Their goal? The survival of the human species.

生き残り

The male reproductive system consists of one group of organs and the female reproductive system consists of another group. These two systems differ in structure, but they share a common function — that of reproducing the human body. We shall discuss the male reproductive system first and then the female reproductive system.

男性の生殖系
女性の生殖系

Human reproduction — ヒトの生殖

Human reproduction differs from reproduction in other animals and in plants because it involves more than just a *biological* (life) process. Among human beings, sex and reproduction may involve love and other deep feelings. Moral standards govern sexual behavior in most societies, and individual members of the societies are expected to follow those standards.

生物学的

道徳的規範

〔出典 B, Vol.16, p.244：R14 〜 R20〕

(1) The male reproductive system — 男性の生殖系

The male *genitals* (sex organs) are mostly outside the body. A man or boy has a finger-shaped organ called a *penis* between his legs. Behind the penis hangs a small sack called the *scrotum*. The scrotum contains two oval-shaped sex organs called *testicles* or

男性生殖器

ペニス〔píːnəs〕

精巣（睾丸, testis の

The Reproductive System

testis. The testicles consist of a complicated system of tubes in which millions of sperm are produced and stored. A tube called the *vas deferens* carries sperm from each testicle to a tube called the *urethra*. A whitish fluid called *semen* is produced by the *prostate gland* and the *seminal vesicles,* and is mixed and stored with the sperm in the vas deferens. The semen, which contains the sperm, is released through the urethra. The urethra runs through the penis. Sperm from the testicles and urine from the bladder are both discharged from the body through the penis, but always at different times.

複数形）
精子
精管
尿道
精液〔síːmən〕, 前立腺

尿, 膀胱

〔出典 B. Vol.16, p.244：R26～p.245：L10〕

(2) The female reproductive system — 女性の生殖系

All the female reproductive organs are inside the body. A woman or girl has small folds of skin called the *vulva* between her legs. The vulva covers the opening to a narrow canal called the *vagina*. The vagina leads to the *uterus*, a hollow, pear-shaped organ. Two organs called *ovaries* produce and store female sex cells. The ovaries lie near the uterus. They are oval-shaped and about the size of a walnut. Normally, the ovaries release one egg about every 28 days in a process called *ovulation*. After ovulation occurs, the egg enters a narrow tube called a *Fallopian tube* or *oviduct*. The Fallopian tubes are not connected to the ovaries, but lie close to them. The tubes carry the eggs to the uterus, which is located between the ovaries.

One of the main differences between the male and

外陰
膣〔vədʒáinə〕
子宮
卵巣

排卵
ファロピオ管, 卵管

(2) The female reproductive system

female reproductive systems involves the way in which sex cells are produced and released. The testicles produce and store millions of sperm that can be released at almost any time. The ovaries produce a few thousand eggs, but only a few hundred of them are released during the female's lifetime. Normally, only one egg at a time is released during ovulation.

The *menstrual cycle* is the process that prepares a woman for pregnancy. During the menstrual cycle, changes take place in the uterus. The soft inner lining of the uterus thickens, reaching its full thickness shortly after ovulation. If the egg is fertilized, it attaches itself to the lining of the uterus and starts to develop. If the egg is not fertilized by a sperm within about 12 hours, it dies. The unfertilized egg, together with the inner lining of the uterus, is then slowly discharged through the vagina in a process called *menstruation*. Menstruation lasts several days. The menstrual cycle repeats itself every 24 to 32 days in most women, unless an egg is fertilized.

月経周期
妊娠

受精する

〔出典 B. Vol.16, p.245：L11 ~ R12〕

Let's pronounce medical English terms.

1. reproductive system
2. genitals
3. sperm
4. ovary

Review questions

1. How does human reproduction differ from one in other animals?
2. In what organ is semen produced and stored?
3. In what organ are female sex cells produced and stored?
4. How long does the egg live?
5. Sort the words below by the female reproductive organs and male repro-

The Reproductive System

ductive ones.
a. ovary   b. penis   c. prostate gland
d. testis   e. seminal vesicle f. uterus
g. vagina   h. vas deferens

Supplementary Reading

The Symposium （饗宴：アリストファネスのことば）

作者：プラトン（427?-?347B.C.），作品出版年：385-380B.C.

あらすじ：この章の Supplementary Reading は，哲学の祖ソクラテスの弟子プラトン（Plato 427?-?347B.C.）の著述 *The Symposium*（饗宴）からの抜粋である．ここには人間の原型について紹介されている．それによると，人間の種類は，男，女，男女（おめ）と3種であって，その姿はすべて球形で，手は4本，足も4本，2つの顔を丸い首の上にもっていた．ところが彼らは神に刃向かったので，ゼウス神（ギリシア神話の最高神）は他の神々と相談して，人間を2つに切断することにした．その結果，人間はかつての半身を求めて探しまわり，出会うと懐しさのあまり抱きあうばかりで，生活に必要なことは何もしないので次第に滅んでいった．ゼウス神は哀れんで（むしろ人間からの貢物が減ると困るので？），彼らの隠し所（reproductive organ）を前に移し，男性によって女性の胎内で生殖を行わせることによって，2つの半身を一体にして人間本来の姿を回復させた……ということである〔出典 L〕．

First of all, you must learn the constitution of man and the modifications which it has undergone, for originally it was different from what it is now.　In the first place there were three sexes, not, as with us, two, male and female; the third partook of the nature of both the others and has vanished, though its name survives.　The hermaphrodite was a distinct sex in form as well as in name, with the characteristics of both male and female, but now the name alone remains, and that solely as a term of abuse.　Secondly, each human being was a rounded whole, with double back and flanks forming a complete circle; it had four hands and an equal number of legs, and two identi-

本性・本質
変形・変化

現在のように男と女の両性だけではなく

両性具有者（男女）

ののしりの言葉

脇腹

cally similar faces upon a circular neck, with one head common to both the faces, which were turned in opposite directions. It had four ears and two organs of generation and everything else to correspond.

These people could walk upright like us in either direction, backwards or forwards, but when they wanted to run quickly they used all their eight limbs, and turned rapidly over and over in a circle, like tumblers who perform a cartwheel and return to an upright position.

The reason for the existence of three sexes and for their being of such a nature is that originally the male sprang from the sun and the female from the earth, while the sex which was both male and female came from the moon, which partakes of the nature of both sun and earth. Their circular shape and their hoop-like method of progression were both due to the fact that they were like their parents. Their strength and vigour made them very formidable, and their pride was overweening; they attacked the gods, and Homer's story of Ephialtes and Otus attempting to climb up to heaven and set upon the gods is related also of these beings.

So Zeus and the other gods debated what was to be done with them. For a long time they were at a loss, unable to bring themselves either to kill them by lightning, as they had the giants, and extinguish the race — thus depriving themselves for ever of the honours and sacrifice due from humanity — or to let them go on in their insolence.

At last, after much painful thought, Zeus had an

まっすぐ立って	
車輪	
輪のような歩き方	
恐るべき	
エピアルテスとオトス	
議論する，（人・問題など）を（どう）始末する	
栄誉	
傲慢	

idea. "I think," he said, "that I have found a way by which we can allow the human race to continue to exist and also put an end to their wickedness by making them weaker. I will cut each of them in two; in this way they will be weaker, and at the same time more profitable to us by being more numerous. They shall walk upright upon two legs. ..." As he bisected each, he bade Apollo turn round the face and the half-neck attached to it towards the cut side, so that the victim, having the evidence of bisection before his eyes, might behave better in future. He also bade him heal the wounds.

半分の頸
犠牲者

So Apollo turned round the faces, and gathering together the skin, like a purse with drawstrings, on to what is now called the belly, he tied it tightly in the middle of the belly round a single aperture which men call the navel. He smoothed out the other wrinkles, which were numerous, and moulded the chest with a tool like those which cobblers use to smooth wrinkles in the leather on their last. But he left a few on the belly itself round the navel, to remind man of the state from which he had fallen. ...

引き締めひもの財布
腹部
開き口
臍
胸を形作る
靴屋

When one member of a pair died and the other was left, the latter sought after and embraced another partner, which might be the half either of a female whole (what is now called a woman) or a male. So they went on perishing till Zeus took pity on them, and hit upon a second plan. He moved their reproductive organs to the front: hitherto they had been placed on the outer side of their bodies, and the processes of begetting and birth had been carried on not

滅び続ける
生殖器

妊娠

The Reproductive System

by the physical union of the sexes, but by emission to the ground, as is the case with grasshoppers. ... His object in making this change was twofold; if male coupled with female, children might be begotten and the race thus continued, but if male coupled with male, at any rate the desire for intercourse would be satisfied, and men set free from it to turn to other activities and to attend to the rest of the business of life.

 It is from this distant epoch, then, that we may date the innate love which human beings feel for one another, the love which restores us to our ancient state by attempting to weld two beings into one and to heal the wounds which humanity suffered.

放出
バッタ・キリギリス

その他の人生の営み

本来の愛

To make sure of your reading.
1. How many beings were there in the beginning of the world according to *The Symposium*?
2. Why did they lose their energy?
3. How did Zeus bring a settlement?

医学英語のルーツ―ギリシア神話（8）
Love（愛）= Psyche（プシュケ）+ Eros（エロス）

　蝶の羽根をもつ美少女がいた．名はプシュケ．彼女が女神のように人々から崇拝されているという噂が，あの美の女神アフロディテをいたく刺激することになった．彼女は，「まー，小娘が．許せません」と気色ばんだこと！怖いのは女の（いえ男もですが）嫉妬である．美しいお顔を歪めて息子のエロス[1]に「あの生意気なプシュケをお前のやじりで射って，さえない男に恋させておしまい」と断固として命じた．

　背中に羽根，手に弓矢をもつ愛の神エロスが矢を射ると，最初に出会った相手が'おかちめんこ'でも，性格が悪くても，どんな相手でも無条件に好きになってしまう．もともと恋とはそういうもの．ほら，昔から"Love is blind."というではないか．

　エロスは，眠っているプシュケにそっと近づきお腹に矢を射った．が，驚いて目覚めたプシュケの美しさにうろたえ，手元がくるって，こともあろうにやじりで自分が怪我してしまったのである．つまり，エロスはプシュケに恋してしまったのだ．でも，神であるエロスの姿は人間には目に見えないために，プシュケはその時は「痛っ」と感じただけ．

　さて，プシュケはアポロンの神託によって「山の頂にいる怪物が夫となるであろう」と運命づけられていた．いつまでも男性に縁のない彼女はとうとう覚悟した．たったひとりで山に向かい，頂に座って怪物を待っていると，ほんわりとやさしい西風が吹いて彼女を抱き抱え，壮麗な宮殿へと連れていった．そして，夜になるとひとりの男性が訪れては，明け方近くになると去っていく．「決して姿を見てはならない，私の愛を疑うな．私はただお前に愛されたいのだ」という言葉に，プシュケは気持ちを抑えて過ごしていた．プシュケの姉二人も美しい女性であったが，女神の嫉妬をかうほどの美しさではなかったからだろうか，早々に結婚していた．ある日妹を久しぶりに訪れた姉たちは，彼女がすばらしい宮殿に住み，夫に愛されていることを知って妬ましくなる．二人して「きっとその人は化け物に違いないわ．だから，姿を見せてくれないのよ」と唆（そそのか）した．

　疑念が生じると耐えられなくなるものである．プシュケはいつものように

漆黒の闇の中をやってきた夫が眠りについた時を見計らうと，灯をともして見た．その顔は，怪物どころか美青年．母の目をすり抜けては逢いにくるエロスだったのだが，約束を破ったプシュケの元を二度と訪れることはなかった．それにしても，エロスはどこででも見えないはずなのに？　それは，さておき……

　エロスに会わせてください，と必死で頼むプシュケにアフロディテは「そうねえ……」と考える振りをし，「私の命じることができたならね」と意地悪な要求をいいつけた．素直で一途なプシュケは，これでもかこれでもかと続く容赦ない命令を何とか果たそうとする．そして不思議なことに，いつも何者かが現れて代わって仕事を終えてくれた．たとえば，いろいろな種類の，しかも気が遠くなるほどの分量の豆を，無数の蟻がやってきて選別してくれる．渦巻く河向こうの金の羊の毛を集めなければならない時には，河の神様が羊をおとなしくさせてくれた（グリム童話の「灰かぶり」によく似た話である）．

　何を命じてもやってのけるプシュケに，アフロディテはとうとう「陰府の国のペルセポネスに美の薬をいくらか分けてもらうよう」と命じた．彼女は底知れない闇の世界をくぐり抜け，やっとの思いで陰府の国にたどりつき，美の妙薬を箱に入れ，再び地上への途についた．箱を開けてはならない，といわれていたのに，プシュケは久しぶりに会うエロスに「きれいだね」とほめてもらいたいと，美をこっそりと分けていただこうかしら，と蓋を開けてしまった．ところが，箱の中には，美の妙薬ではなく「冥界の眠り」があった．もやもやと溢れ出た眠りのもとを浴びて，彼女はその場で前後不覚になってしまった．心配と逢いたさで待ちきれずに飛んできたエロスが大急ぎで眠りを集め箱に収めたので，プシュケはようやく目を覚ますことができたのである（実は睡眠が美の妙薬？）．

　さて少々マザコン気味のエロスだが，今度ばかりは母の妨害を恐れずゼウス神に懸命にお願いをしたので，ゼウスはアフロディテに「二人を一緒にさせてやろう」と仲介の労をとった．いいところもあるではないか．ゼウスはプシュケに不老不死のお酒を飲ませて女神に変身させ，二人は遂に神々公認の夫婦になることができた．そして，二人の間に「喜び」が生まれたという．めでたし，めでたし．

Psyche と Eros に因む医学英語

psychiatry　精神医学：psychology との違いは，-iatro（iatros = 医師）が語に含まれていることで識別できる．

psychology　心理学：-logy（学問）

psychoanalysis　精神分析（学）

psychopathy　精神病：-pathy（病気．語源は pathos（苦しみ）である）

psychosomatic disease　心身症

eros　エロス，生の本能（精神分析で，生殖，生命に向かう本能を表す生命原理）

eroticism　好色症

erotopathy　性倒錯

erotophobia　色情恐怖症

aphrodisiac　性欲亢進（とくに過度の場合）．aphro- は泡の意味．

CHAPTER 13
Aging and the end of life
加齢と生の終焉

Aging — 加齢

    Aging is the process of growing old. Most living things undergo two basic types of biological change during their lifetime. One is growth, an increase in the size or efficiency of an organism. The other is aging, which involves a decrease or leveling off in size or efficiency. Growth and aging can occur at the same time.

    Signs of aging begin to appear in most people between the age of 30 and 40. Heredity determines most of the ways a person changes while aging, but environment also plays a role.

    Graying hair is probably the most common sign of aging. Another is *arcus senilis*, a cloudy ring that forms around the cornea of the eye. All the senses decline with age. For example, the eyes lose their ability to adapt to darkness, and they require brighter light for reading. The lens of the eye cannot adjust so well as before to near and distant vision. A person also loses the ability to hear sounds of high frequency. About half the taste buds may be lost, and the capaci-

老化
受ける
成長
有効性

老化の徴候
遺伝形質

環境
白髪
老人環
角膜

水晶体

高周波
味蕾

154

ty to detect odors decreases greatly.

Movement also becomes more difficult with age. By the age of 80, about half the muscle cells have been replaced by other kinds of tissue. A connective material, composed largely of a protein called *collagen*, occupies the space between cells. Aging makes strands of collagen link together and become less elastic. In women especially, the bones lose calcium and become more likely to break.

As a person ages, the body's ability to combat infection declines. This change occurs because the white blood cells of what is called the body's *immune system* lose their protective function.

Many people believe that with advancing age, an individual loses the ability to learn, remember, and make decisions. But unless disease or injury damages the brain, a healthy elderly person who remains physically and mentally active probably suffers no serious decline in mental capacity.

Scientists distinguish between two types of aging. *Primary aging*, also called *senescence*, includes the unavoidable changes in the structure and composition of the body that are determined by heredity. *Secondary aging* includes disabilities caused by illness or accidental damage. Most serious changes associated with old age result from secondary aging.

The branch of medicine that deals with the diseases of old age is called *geriatrics*. The study of the aging process itself is known as *gerontology*.

No one completely understands the aging process. Some scientists doubt that human aging will ever be

Aging and the end of life

controlled.　Others believe that aging can be conquered.　They note that several species of fish continue to grow until death, without ever appearing to age. Also, single-celled animals seem to lose all signs of age after each of the many times they reproduce.　　　　生殖する

Normal human cells can be kept alive in a laboratory for only a limited time.　But abnormal cells, such as various kinds of cancer cells, can be sustained indefinitely.　If scientists can determine how such abnormal cells survive, they may gain an insight into the process of cell aging.

実験室

異常細胞

[出典 B, Vol.1, p.142: L38 ~ R36]

| Let's pronounce medical English terms. |

1. heredity　　2. arcus senilis　　3. collagen
4. geriatrics　　5. gerontology

| Review questions |

1. What biological changes do most living things undergo in their lifetime?
2. What are the signs of aging?
3. Explain briefly the difference between geriatrics and gerontology.
4. How can we overcome our aging?
5. Find the appropriate definition for each word.
   1) heredity　　　　(　　　　)
   2) collagen　　　　(　　　　)
   3) geriatrics　　　(　　　　)
   4) gerontology　　(　　　　)
   5) senescence　　 (　　　　)
   a. the scientific study of old age, the process of aging, and the particular problems of old people
   b. the branch of medicine or social science dealing with the health and care of old people
   c. the process of becoming old and showing the effects of being old age
   d. bundles of protein fibers, which form the connective tissue, bone

and cartilage
e. the process by which mental and physical characteristics are passed by parents to their children

Aging and the end of life

Death — 死

Death is the end of life. Every living thing eventually dies, but human beings are probably the only creatures that can imagine their own deaths. | いずれは
| 生物

Most people fear death and try to avoid thinking about it. However, people's awareness of death has been one of the chief forces in the development of civilization. Throughout history, people have continually sought new medical knowledge with which to delay death. Philosophers and religious leaders have tried to understand the meaning of death. Some scholars believe that much human progress results from people's efforts to overcome death and gain immortality through lasting achievements. | 考えることを避けようとする 死の自覚 文明の発達 延ばす 哲学者と宗教指導者 学者 不死を獲得する

(1) Medical aspects of death — 死の医学的側面

Scientists recognize three types of death that occur during the life of all organisms except those consisting of only one cell. These types are *necrobiosis, necrosis,* and somatic death. | 有機体 類壊死, 壊死 身体死

Necrobiosis is the continual death and replacement of individual cells through life. Except for nerve cells, all the cells of an organism are constantly being replaced. For example, new skin cells form under the surface as the old ones die and flake off. | はがれ落ちる

Necrosis is the death of tissues or even entire organs. During a heart attack, for example, a blood clot cuts off the circulation of the blood to part of the heart. The affected part dies, but the organism continues to live unless the damage has been severe. | 心臓発作, 血液凝固 損傷

Somatic death is the end of all life processes in an

organism. A person whose heart and lungs stop working may be considered *clinically dead*, but somatic death may not yet have occurred. The individual cells of the body continue to live for several minutes. The person may be revived if the heart and lungs start working again and give the cells the oxygen they need. After about three minutes, the brain cells — which are most sensitive to a lack of oxygen — begin to die. The person is soon dead beyond any possibility of revival. Gradually, other cells of the body also die. The last ones to perish are the bone, hair, and skin cells, which may continue to grow for several hours.

Many changes take place after death. The temperature of the body slowly drops to that of its surroundings. The muscles develop a stiffening called *rigor mortis*. The blood, which no longer circulates, settles and produces reddish-purple discolorations in the lowest areas of the body. Eventually, bacteria and other tiny organisms grow on the corpse and cause it to decay.

(2) Defining death ― 死の定義

Traditionally, a person whose breathing and heartbeat had stopped was considered dead. Today, however, physicians can prolong the functioning of the lungs and heart by artificial means. Various machines can produce breathing and a heartbeat even in a patient whose brain has been destroyed. These new medical procedures have led many physicians, lawyers, and religious leaders to favor a new definition of death called *brain death*. Under this definition, a

臨床的死
個々の細胞

生き返る

…に最も敏感な
回復の可能性

死ぬ

体温

死後硬直

赤紫色の変色

死体

呼吸, 脈

引き延ばす
人工的手段

医学的手順

脳死

person is considered dead if a device called an *electroencephalograph* detects no brain activity for at least 24 hours. The individual's circulation and breathing may be maintained by machine during that period.

The brain-death definition of death raises important medical, legal, and moral questions. People who support this definition argue that it benefits society by making vital organs available for transplants. In most cases, the organs of a person who is dead under the traditional definition cannot be transplanted. But many vital organs remain alive and functioning in an individual whose body processes are maintained by machine, even though brain activity has stopped. Physicians can remove these organs and use them in transplants — if brain death is accepted as a legal definition.

Critics of the brain-death definition point out that there are many unanswered questions regarding this concept. Such questions include: Who should decide which definition of death to use? When has brain death reached the point where it cannot be reversed?

(3) The right to die — 死ぬ権利

Many people believe that physicians should use every means to maintain a person's life as long as possible. But others argue that dying patients and their physicians have the right to choose whether life-maintaining treatments should be continued. Some people also feel that this decision should be left to the family and physician if the patient is no longer capable of expressing his or her wishes. People who hold

(3) The right to die

these attitudes contend that physicians are not obligated to provide treatment that would only temporarily extend the life of a hopelessly ill or injured person.

 Some people believe that hopelessly ill patients should not only have the right to refuse treatment, but also to be put painlessly to death if they desire. They contend that each person has the right to control his or her life and to determine the time of his or her death. Others maintain that this right should be extended to the family of dying patients who are no longer capable of expressing their own desires. In these cases, they argue, the family and physician should be permitted to painlessly end the patient's suffering. Putting hopelessly ill persons to death — with or without their requesting it — is called *euthanasia*, or *mercy killing*. Euthanasia is illegal in the United States, Canada, and almost all other countries.

回復の望みのない病気にかかった，または負傷した人

患者の苦痛

〔jùːθənéɪʒ(i)ə〕
安楽死，違法な
［出 典 B, Vol.5, p.60: R18 ～ p.61: L61］

| Let's pronounce medical English terms. |

1. immortality   2. necrobiosis   3. necrosis
4. somatic death   5. corpse   6. euthanasia

| Review questions |

1. Describe briefly three scientific types of death.
2. What definition was considered traditionally as an individual death?
3. Explain the reason why the definition of brain death has been raised.
4. Is 'euthanasia' legal in Japan?
5. Put the following English into Japanese.
　1) immortality   (　　　　)
　2) necrosis   (　　　　)
　3) somatic death   (　　　　)
　4) brain death   (　　　　)

Aging and the end of life

5) euthanasia (   )

医学英語の常識（10）
What is human? —語源から導かれること

英語の human は，その語源を homō（ギリシア語の「同じ」，ラテン語の「人間」という意味）から派生した hūmānus にまで逆のぼる．そこから古期フランス語 humain へ，そして中期英語 humayne が humane となり，18世紀の初めごろ，現代英語の human というつづりになった．

homó は，土・大地という意味のラテン語 humus と語根を同じくする．面白いことに humble（謙遜な）の語根も humus だが，その語根はラテン語の humilis（低いという意味）である．これまでに「医学英語のルーツ」で何度か登場したギリシア神話の女神ガイア（Gaia）はギリシア語で「土地，地球」という意味である．ヘブライ語では，聖書に登場する人類最初の人間アダムを Ādām といい，それは "adāmā（土）より造られし者" という意味の háádam から名づけられたのである．旧約聖書 "創世記" にも，人は土から造られ（創世記2章7節），汗して土を耕し食物を栽培し，そしてついには土に還る（創世記3章19節）と記述されている．

このように，古代人がいだいた人間のイメージは，かぎりなく土に近い存在であったといえる．にもかかわらず，バベルの人々が天まで届く塔を建設しようと試みた時，神からその塔を壊され，共通の言語を奪われてしまった（創世記11章1-9節）姿は，どことなく現代の人々の姿と重複する気がしないでもない．

20世紀に，医学は機械器具の発達に伴って急速に進歩した．その結果，人を眠ったまま生かすことも，他の人間の臓器を譲り受けることも可能にした．21世紀に入るとヒトの皮膚から万能細胞を作ることも可能になった．それが崩れ落ちてしまうバベルの塔にならないように心し，human であり，homo sapience（知恵ある人）であろうとすることが，医学・医療に携わる者の務めであろうと思われる．

Aging and the end of life

Supplementary Reading

Consideration on NARAYAMA-Song
(楢山節考)

作者：深沢七郎（1914-1981），作品出版年：1956
あらすじ：「楢山節考」は，今昔物語からのいい伝えをもとに書かれた深沢七郎の中編小説である．

　山深い'おりん'の村では，食いぶちを減らすために70歳になると死出の旅（楢山参り）に向かう，という掟があった．おりんは数年前から別れの宴で村人に振る舞う白萩（コメの飯），白酒を準備し，楢山で座る筵を織り，息子の辰平の後妻を探し，その嫁に貴重なヤマメの取り方を教えた．そしてきっぱりと死を受け入れ，息子に背負われて楢山へと向かう．辰平が楢山におりんを置き山道を降りていくと，雪が舞い始める．彼は決して戻ってはならないという山の掟を破って駆けもどり，"How wonderful it is that it's snowing!"と母親に声をかける．生きることが困難であった時代に人の情を通い合わせる人々の姿に感動さえ覚える読者は多いであろう〔出典M，英訳：清水雅子〕．

Before O'Rin's Pilgrimage to NARAYAMA ―楢山参りの前に

　Mountains ranging over mountains, there is nothing but mountains as far as the eye can see.　Amidst these mountains in Shinshu, the house of O'Rin stood at the edge of the village, "Muko-mura", which means, the village beyond the mountains. ...　O'Rin had come here as a bride fifty years before.

　O'Rin was now sixty-nine years old, and her husband had died more than twenty years before. The wife of Tatsuhei, her only son, had also died when, on her way to pick chestnuts, she had rolled down into a ravine.　The worry about seeking a second wife for

山また山が連なって
只中に
おりん
向こう村

栗ノ山峡

him was greater than looking after her four grandchildren, because a suitable widow was not to be found anywhere in the village nor in the "village over there". ...

 寡婦

For a long time, O'Rin had been determined to go on a pilgrimage to Narayama. She had already prepared "sake" for a farewell feast. Three years before she had already prepared a mat, on which she would sit when she arrived at the mountain. Last, but not least, a second wife for her widowed Tatsuhei had to be found. Now all was finished: the sake, the mat, and the daughter-in-law. Nevertheless she still had one more thing to settle.

 楢山参り

 筵（むしろ）

After O'Rin made sure that nobody was around, she took up a flint. She struck herself — bang! bang! — on the upper and lower anterior teeth with it. In this way, she tried smash her solid teeth with it. It was terrible pain, which roared through her she had to become ashamed of them after all. While her son, Tatsuhei, had already lost a considerable number of his teeth, O'Rin's full set aroused an impression, as if she could devour anything at all. One had to be ashamed of such teeth in a village where there was not enough food for everyone.

 火打石
 前歯

 完全に揃った歯
 むさぼり合う

To NARAYAMA — 楢山へ

One night later on, O'Rin forced the irresolute Tatsuhei to depart and begin her pilgrimage to Narayama. In the evening she had already washed the "Shira Hagi" which was to be eaten the following day and had told Tama-yan how to find fungi and to capture

 気が進まない

 白萩さま＝白いご飯

 玉やん（辰平の嫁），

Aging and the end of life

trout. After she made sure that all the people in the house were asleep, she went silently through the doorway to the backward. There she climbed on carrying board which Tatsuhei had strapped to his back. It was a windless but icy cold night. As the sky was overcast, the moon was not visible and Tatsuhei walked on the path unsteadily. After O'Rin and Tatsuhei had gone out, Tama-yan slipped out of her bed. She opened the door and went out. Leaning one hand on the trunk of the tree, she peered into the darkness and watched as the two slipped into the night.

As he climbed higher and higher, nothing but oaks was seen. Finally he came to a spot which looked like the summit. At the foot of a big boulder by which he passed, he happened to notice something. Tatsuhei jumped back involuntarily. The person learning against the base of the rock was a corpse. It had clenched both fists and seemed to press them against each other. Tatsuhei came to a standstill, frozen by the sight. O'Rin swung her arms back and forth motioning him to continue onward.

The path continued to climb. Several steps further on, ... O'Rin struck him on the shoulder, and kicked him with her legs. She wanted him to let her down from the carrying board on his back. Tatsuhei slipped off the board. When she got down, she spread out the mat which she had carried tied around her waist.

O'Rin stood bolt upright on the mat. ... O'Rin's hands gripped him tightly. Then she pushed him vigorously on the back. Tatsuhei left. He kept walk-

きのこ，岩魚

笈（おいこ）

樫の木

山頂，大きな岩

死体

ing without turning around keeping the vow of the mountain. 誓い

He kept on until he was about halfway down Narayama when he noticed something white. He stopped and looked into the distance. In the middle of the oaks, like white dust, snow was dancing. "Ah!" Tatsuhei exclaimed. He greedily stared at the snow, which had grown into a storm. What O'Rin had always proclaimed with pride, had come true. 白い粉のように / 断言する

By the time he reached the boulder behind which O'Rin was sitting, the snow had completely covered the ground. Not only was he breaking the vow of pilgrimage to the mountain by returning back, but he also was going to break the vow by speaking to her. That corresponded to a crime. But, just as she had said "It will surely snow!" it had begun to snow. That was the one word that he wanted to tell her. 話しかける / 罪に相当する

Tatsuhei said loudly, "Mama, it's snowing."

Slowly O'Rin swung her hand in the down-the-mountain direction. "Go home! Go home!" she seemed to say. 山の下の方へ

"Mama, you will freeze!" ... "How wonderful it is that it's snowing!" One is less likely to freeze, when one is wrapped with snow, than when one is exposed to the cold mountain air, he thought, "In this way Mama will simply fall asleep in the end." 凍える / 〜に曝される

"Mama, you are lucky, it's snowing!" Then he spoke the words of the song to himself, "On the day when she goes into the mountain. ..."

O'Rin inclined her head approvingly but again gestured in the direction of home. Tatsuhei shouted, わかったというように

Aging and the end of life

"Mama, it's really snowing!" and ran down the mountain like a fleeing hare.   　　　　　足のすばやい兎

To make sure of your reading.
1. Did O'Rin and other members of her family have enough foods?
2. What is the most worry for O'Rin before her going to Narayama?
3. What did O'Rin prepare before going to Narayama?
4. Why did Tatsuhei return back to O'Rin when it began to snow?

医学英語のルーツ―ギリシア神話 (9)
Man is mortal ― 永遠の眠りの神タナトス (Tanatos) を受容するということ

　人は'死すべきもの (mortal)'であるがゆえに，昔から不老・不死を願ってきた．ギリシア神話では，人間を超えて容姿の美しいエンデュミオンが，生きて老いて美を失うよりも，美しいままで永遠の眠りにつくことを選んだという．また女神エーオスはトロイ王の息子，人間ティートノスとの恋を永遠にするためにゼウス神に彼の不死を願う．ところが不老を願うことを忘れたため，彼は年老いて青年のころの輝くような美しさを失っていった．エーオスは見るにみかねて彼を一室に閉じ込めてしまう．死ぬこともできず老い続けたティートノスは，最後は蝉（一説ではコオロギ）になってしまった，と神話は伝える．

　話が前後するが，ギリシア神話では「タナトス」は人間のかぎりある生の最期，「ジェラス」(Geras) はそれ以前の私たちの人生の最後の日々を象徴する神々である．死の神タナトスは，夜になると弟ヒュプノスを連れて地上に現れる．私たちは毎夜，優しい眠りの神のお蔭で一日の労苦を忘れ，ひとときの安らぎを得ることができるのだ．しかしやがて，ジェラス（老い）が私たちのもとを訪れ，タナトスが容赦なく永遠の眠りを運命づける．そもそもタナトスのみが人間に死を与える存在ではない．人間は生まれた時にすでに死ぬ運命にある．なぜなら，人の寿命は三人の運命の女神モイライ (Moirai) ― 生命の糸の紡ぎ手（クロト）・配り手（ラクシス）・切り手（アトポロス）― によって定められており，あのゼウスやアテナでさえも，変更させるのは不可能に近い．

　かつて日本においても老いと死は深刻な問題であった．今昔物語に書かれた棄老をモチーフにした「楢山節考」が出版されたのは，日本が戦争による荒廃から立ち直り，高度成長期に入ろうとした昭和31年であった．経済的に豊かになりつつあった日本の人々に，老いと死はいつの時代にも変わらない重いテーマであると強烈に印象づけたのであった．

　戦後，日本人の平均寿命は伸び続け，今や世界一の高齢社会となった．しかし，それは必ずしも人が元気で生きる生活を保障するという意味ではない．

Aging and the end of life

100歳を超えてなお，かくしゃくとして人生を楽しむ高齢者の姿に，逆に私たちが励まされる場合もあるが，高齢期が長くなるのは'恍惚の人'となる可能性を含み，経済的な不安も重なって高齢者の'老い'への不安は増している．そして現代では「楢山節考」の'おりん'のように掟によって死出の旅に向かうことはないものの，施設でも，あるいは自宅でも，ひとりぼっちで現代版楢山というべき状況の中で人生を終える人々は増加の一途をたどっている．私たちは，高齢者が人生の馳せ場を無事に駆け抜けるには，どのようなサポートができるのだろうか？

昔も今も，人は必ず死ぬと知っており，人生における諸々の出来事のうち，これほど確実な予定は見あたりそうにない．けれども，どのように死ぬかということはまったく知らされていないのである．だからこそ，人は日ごろから自らの死を準備する気構えをもち，自らを教育する必要があろう．ローマの教育者セネカ曰く，「不思議なことに，一生をかけて学ぶべきは，死ぬことである」．

Tanatos と Geras に因む医学英語

euthanasia 安楽死（eu- は「よい」という意味）
thanatology 死の心理学，死相論（死の研究に関する学問）
thanatophobia 死恐怖症
atropine アトロピン（痙攣緩和薬．Atropos に因む．ナス科植物から得られる有毒のアルカロイド）
gerontology 老年学（加齢・老人問題を研究する学問）
gerontoxon 老人環 = arcus senilis（眼の角膜内の脂肪顆粒の沈着）
geriatrics 老年（老人）医学（老年者の医療に関する医学）．-iatro-（iatrikos）は治療者（医師）にかかわる用語をつくる．

Appendix

Planes and directions　断面と方向

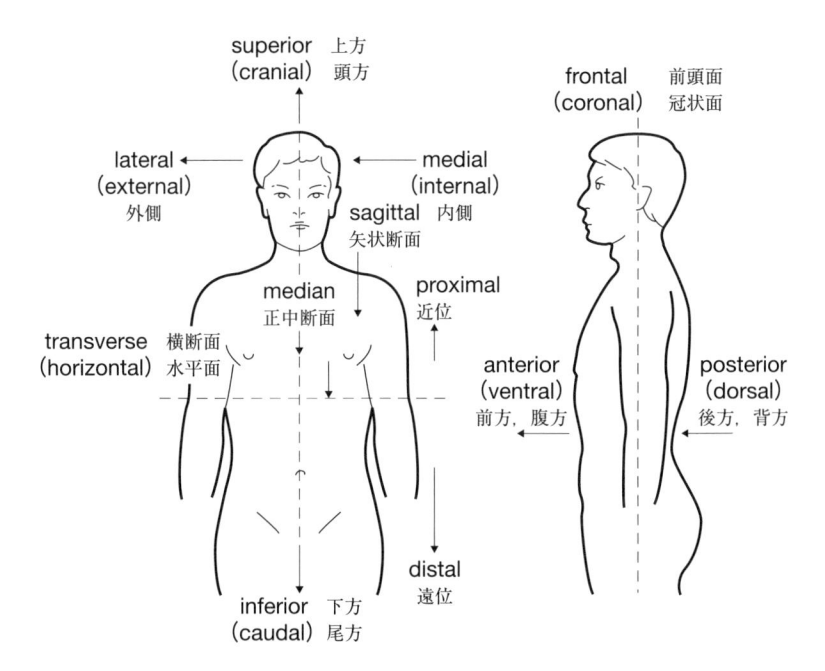

- superior (cranial)　上方　頭方
- lateral (external)　外側
- medial (internal)　内側
- sagittal　矢状断面
- median　正中断面
- proximal　近位
- transverse (horizontal)　横断面　水平面
- distal　遠位
- inferior (caudal)　下方　尾方
- frontal (coronal)　前頭面　冠状面
- anterior (ventral)　前方，腹方
- posterior (dorsal)　後方，背方

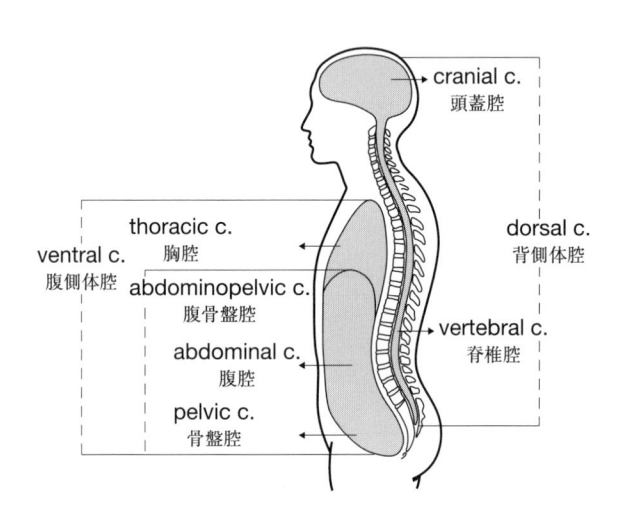

Appendix

```
                    cranial c.
                    頭蓋腔

        thoracic c.
        胸腔
ventral c.                      dorsal c.
腹側体腔                         背側体腔
        abdominopelvic c.
        腹骨盤腔
                                vertebral c.
        abdominal c.            脊椎腔
        腹腔

        pelvic c.
        骨盤腔
```

Cavities of the body　体腔

dorsal cavity　背側体腔
　　cranial c.　頭蓋腔
　　vertebral c.　脊椎腔（spinal cord　脊髄）
ventral cavity　腹側体腔
　　thoracic c.　胸腔（lungs　肺, mediastinum　縦隔構造, heart　心臓）
　　abdominopelvic c.　腹骨盤腔
　　　　abdominal c.　腹腔（liver　肝臓, gallbladder　胆のう, stomach　胃, spleen　脾臓,
　　　　　　　　　　　　pancreas　膵臓, small intestine　小腸, large intestine　大腸）
　　　　pelvic c.　骨盤腔（urinary bladder　膀胱, sigmoid colon　S字結腸, rectum　直腸,
　　　　　　　　　　　　reproductive organ　生殖器官）

注）（　）は含まれる器官, 組織. the は省略. c. = cavity

172

Terms for hospital（病院用語）

station	部署	treatment room	治療室
stethoscope	聴診器	emergency clinic room	救急外来室
bandage	包帯	infection isolation room	感染隔離室
absorbent cotton	脱脂綿	clinical laboratory	臨床検査室
gauze	ガーゼ	blood laboratory	血液尿検査室
sticking plaster	絆創膏	radiology laboratory (X-ray room)	X線撮影室
basin	洗面器		
ice bag	氷のう	ultrasound laboratory	超音波検査室
hypodermic needle	注射針	renal hemodialysis laboratory (room)	腎透析室
clinical thermometer	体温計		
surgical knife, scalpel	メス	treadmill stress test laboratory	心臓負荷検査室
test tube	試験管		
blood pressure gauge, sphygmomanometer	血圧計	rehabilitation center	リハビリテーションセンター
instillator	点滴	helicopter landing place	ヘリポート
giving set	点滴セット	autopsy room	死体解剖室
cast（英）,	ギプス	wards	病棟
plaster（米）		hospice ward	ホスピス病棟
crutch	松葉杖	sickroom	病室
chart, notes	カルテ	nurse center	看護師詰所
prescription	処方	operating room（米）, operating theatre（英）	手術室
first aid	応急処置		
ambulance	救急車	delivery room	分娩室
(wheeled) stretcher	担架	dispensary	薬局
information desk	受付	outpatient clinic	外来
waiting room	待合室	admissions department	入退院センター
examination room	診察室		

Medical staff

hospital administrator	病院長	medical technologist	臨床検査技師
doctor	医師	（米）medical technologist	臨床検査技師（学士号）
physician	内科医		
director of nursing supervisor	看護師長 管理部長	（米）laboratory technician	臨床検査技師
head nurse	病棟看護師主任	radiographic technologist	放射線技師
registered nurse	（正）看護師	（米）radiographer	放射線診断技師
practical nurse	准看護師	（米）radiology technician	放射線治療技師
midwife	助産師		
public health nurse	保健師	（米）nuclear medicine technologist	核医学技師
school nurse	学校看護師		
general practitioner	開業医	dietitian	管理栄養士

Appendix

dietetic technician	栄養士	pharmacist	薬剤師
nutritionist	栄養士, 栄養学者	speech therapist	言語聴覚士
dental hygienist	歯科衛生士	oculometric technician	視力検査士
dental laboratory technician	歯科技工士	record librarian	病歴士
medical engineer	医用工学士	medical social worker	医療ソーシャルワーカー
physical therapist	理学療法士	psychiatric social worker	精神保健福祉士
occupational therapist	作業療法士		
internal medicine	→ physician, internist		内科（医）
surgery	→ surgeon		外科
cardiac surgery			心臓外科
thoracic surgery			胸部外科
orthopedics	→ orthopedist		整形外科
plastic surgery			形成外科
pediatrics	→ pediatrician, child doctor		小児科
ophthalmology	→ ophthalmologist, eye doctor		眼科
otolaryngology, otorhinolaryngology	→ otolaryngologist, nose and throat doctor		耳鼻咽喉科
dermatology	→ dermatologist		皮膚科
neurology	→ neurologist		神経科
psychiatry	→ psychiatrist, clinical psychologist, psychotherapist		精神科
obstetrics	→ obstetrician		産科
gyn(a)ecology	→ gynecologist		婦人科
radiology	→ radiologist		放射線科
anaesthesiology	→ anaesthesiologist		麻酔科
proctology	→ proctologist		肛門科
odontology	→ odontologist		歯科学
dentistry	→ dentist		歯科
urology	→ urologist		泌尿器科

Others（その他）

allergy & immunology	アレルギー・免疫学	mycology	真菌学
		nephrology	腎臓病学
anatomy	解剖学	pathology	病理学
endocrinology	内分泌学	physiology	生理学
hematology	血液学		

Education（教育）

professional course	専門教育	qualification examination	資格試験
clinical practice	臨床実習	governmental examination	国家試験

Names of diseases（病名）

General disease（一般的な病名）

cataract	白内障	heart failure	心不全
glaucoma	緑内障	myocardial infarction	心筋梗塞症
keratoconjunctivitis	角結膜炎	arteriosclerosis	動脈硬化症
eye strain, asthenopia	眼精疲労	cerebral apoplexy	脳卒中
nose bleed	鼻血	anemia	貧血
allergic rhinitis (pollenosis)	アレルギー性鼻炎（花粉症）	hypertension	高血圧
		hypotension	低血圧
otitis media	中耳炎	asthma	ぜんそく
stomatitis	口内炎	obesity	肥満
constipation	便秘	burn	やけど
chronic constipation	慢性便秘	sunstroke (heliosis)	日射病
diarrhea	下痢	insomnia	不眠症
anal fistula	痔瘻	gout	痛風
sciatica	坐骨神経痛	dislocation	脱臼
low back pain	腰痛	sprain (stremma)	捻挫
appendicitis	虫垂炎	abortion	流産
gastric ulcer	胃潰瘍	gestosis	妊娠中毒症
hepatitis	肝炎	morning sickness	つわり
diabetes	糖尿病	hysteromyoma	子宮筋腫
cancer, carcinoma	癌	depression	うつ
tumor	腫瘍	senile dementia	老年性痴呆
ulcer	潰瘍	climacteric disturbance	更年期障害
polyp	ポリープ	food poisoning	食中毒

acute disease（急性疾患）

acute abdomen	急性腹痛
—— alcoholism	——アルコール中毒
—— bronchitis	——気管支炎
—— disseminated encephalomyelitis	——散在性脳脊髄炎
—— hepatitis	——肝炎
—— otitis media	——中耳炎
—— rhinitis	——鼻炎
—— pharyngitis	——咽頭炎（のどかぜ）
—— pyogenic osteomyelitis	——化膿性骨髄炎
—— tonsillitis	——扁桃炎

chronic disease（慢性疾患）

chronic alcoholism	慢性アルコール中毒（アルコール依存症）
—— adrenal cortical insufficiency	——副腎皮質不全
—— enteritis	——腸炎
—— gastritis	——胃炎
—— inflammation of paranasal sinuses	——副鼻腔炎（蓄膿症）
—— pancreatitis	——膵炎
—— renal failure	——腎不全
—— articular rheumatism	——関節リューマチ
—— subdural hematoma	——硬膜下血腫
—— thyroiditis	——甲状腺炎

Appendix

subacute	亜急性	sudden	突発性
contagious	伝染性	protopathic	原発性
infectious	感染(伝染)性	congenital	先天性
epidemic	流行性	acquired	後天性
allergic	アレルギー性	constitutional	体質性
irritable	過敏性	pernicious, malignant	悪性
bacterial	細菌性	benign, benignant	良性
primary	原発性		

Contagious disease (伝染性疾患)

chicken pox	水ぼうそう	pneumonia	肺炎
cholera	コレラ	polio (poliomyelitis)	ポリオ(灰白髄炎)
diphtheria	ジフテリア		
dysentery	赤痢	rubella	風疹
measles(複数形)	麻疹(はしか)	whooping cough	百日咳
mumps(複数形)	おたふくかぜ		

Symptom (病気の兆候)

diarrhea	下痢	convulsion	痙攣
paralysis, palsy	麻痺	fit	ひきつけ／発作
fever	熱	spasm	痙攣
pricky heat	あせも(紅色汗疹)	drug eruption	薬疹
		rash	発疹
eczema	湿疹	malnutrition	栄養不良
vomiting	嘔吐	yawn	あくび
nausea	吐き気		

注)symptom：患者が経験する，あるいは病気が示す構造，機能，あるいは感覚における病的徴候または正常外の逸脱・疾病，主観的徴候．
　　sign：医師の所見における何らかの疾病を示唆する異常・疾病の客観的徴候．

Expression of wound, etc. (傷の表現)

wound	武器による傷	punctured wound	刺し傷
injury	負傷	bruise	打撲傷
cut	切り傷	scratch	ひっかき傷
slash	刃物傷	scrape	すり傷
gash	深い傷	abrasion	すりむき傷
slight (shallow) wound	浅い傷	scar	傷あと
serious (severe) wound	重い傷		

Types of medicine（薬の種類）

oral medicine（経口薬）

tablet	錠剤	pill	丸剤
capsule	カプセル剤	liquid medicine	水薬
powder	散剤	granule	顆粒

application（外用薬）

ointment, salve	軟膏剤	suppository, bougie	坐剤
liniment	リニメント，塗布剤	eyedrops	点眼薬（目薬）
		nosedrops	点鼻薬
poultice	湿布薬	gargle, mouthwash	うがい薬
inhalant	吸入薬		

anesthetic（麻酔薬）

general a.	全身——	peridural a.	硬膜下——
topical a.	局所——	intranasal a.	鼻腔内——
spinal a.	脊椎——		

medicine by the effectiveness（薬効別）

tranquilizer	トランキライザー（精神安定剤）	lozenge	せき止めシロップ
		laxative	下剤
antihistamine	抗ヒスタミン剤	clysma	浣腸剤
antibiotics	抗生物質	coloclysis	浣腸
antidote	解毒剤	cardiotonic, digitalis	強心剤，ジギタリス
anticarcinogen, carcinostatic	抗癌剤	sedative	鎮静剤
insulin	インスリン	vitamins	ビタミン剤
antifebrile	解熱剤	Chinese herbal medicine, kanpo	漢方薬
aspirin	アスピリン（鎮痛，解熱抗炎症薬）	antihypertensive agent	降圧剤
		antiulcerative	抗潰瘍薬
cold medicine	風邪薬	antiphlogistic	消炎剤
cough medicine	せき止め	disinfectant	抗菌剤

Appendix

Terms of examination (検査用語)

X-ray examination	X線検査
direct radiography	直接撮影
indirect radiography (fluorography)	間接撮影
serial radiography	連続撮影
angiography	血管造影法
radioisotope scintigraphy examination	シンチグラフィー検査(RI検査)
chest X-ray	胸部撮影(造影)
abdominal X-ray	腹部撮影(造影)
mammography	乳房撮影(造影)
kidney, ureter, bladder X-ray (KUB)	腎,尿管,膀胱X線撮影(造影)
urethrocystography (UCG)	尿道,膀胱撮影(造影)
cystography	膀胱撮影(造影)
pyelography	腎盂撮影(造影)
cholecystography	胆のう撮影(造影)
cerebral ventriculography	脳室撮影(造影)
bronchography	気管支撮影(造影)
nephrography	腎撮影(造影)
angiocardiography	血管心臓造影法
coronary angiography	冠動脈血管造影法
left ventriculography (LVG)	左心室血管造影法
cerebral angiography	脳血管造影法
aortography	大動脈造影法
carotid angiography (CAG)	頸動脈造影法
magnetic resonance imaging (MRI)	磁気共鳴血管造影法
endoscopy	内視鏡検査
endoscopic pancreatocholangiography	内視鏡的膵胆管造影法
bronchoscopy	気管支鏡検査
esophagoscopy	食道鏡検査
laryngoscopy	咽頭鏡検査
peritoneoscopy	腹腔鏡検査
cystoscopy	膀胱鏡検査
proctoscopy	直腸鏡検査
gastrocamera	胃カメラ
gastro-intestinal series (G-I series)/ Magen-Durch-Leuchtung (MDL)	胃透視
upper G-I	胃・十二指腸・食道透視
lower G-I	空腸以下透視
radioimmunoassay (RIA)	ラジオイムノアッセイ(放射免疫測定法)
scintigraphy	シンチグラフィー
radioisotope imaging	ラジオアイソトープイメージング
computed tomography (CT)	コンピュータ断層撮影法

brain CT (CT of the head)	頭部 CT
thoracal CT (chest CT)	胸部 CT
abdominal CT	腹部 CT
emission computed tomography (ECT)	放射型コンピュータ断層撮影
computerized axial tomography (CTT, CAT)	X線体軸断層撮影
radionuclide computed tomography (RCT)	放射性核種コンピュータ断層撮影
posistron emission tomography (PET)	陽電子放射型断層撮影(法)

Other examinations（その他の検査）

ultrasonic examination	超音波検査
ophthalmotonometry	眼圧測定法
electrocardiography (ECG, EKG)	心電図検査
electroencephalography (EEG)	脳波検査
pulmonaryfunction test	肺機能検査
audiometry	聴力検査
eyesight test	視力検査
blood test	血液検査
urine test	尿検査
biopsy	生検
vaginal smear test	腟スミア診

Appendix

Common medical abbreviations（略語）

abdo (abd)	abdomen	腹部
ACTH	adrenocorticotrophic hormone	副腎皮質刺激ホルモン
ADL	activities of daily living	日常生活動作
AH	acute hepatitis	急性肝炎
AI	aortic incompetence; artificial insemination	大動脈弁閉鎖不全；人工授精
ALP	alkaline phosphatase	アルカリフォスファターゼ
AIDS	acquired immunodeficiency syndrome	後天性免疫不全症候群
ALL	acute lymphocytic leukemia	急性リンパ性白血病
ALS	amyotrophic lateral sclerosis	筋萎縮性側索硬化症
ALT (GPT)	alanine aminotransferase (glutamic pyruvic transaminase)	アラニンアミノトランスフェーゼ（グルタミン酸ピルビン酸トランスアミナーゼ）
AST (GOT)	aspartate aminotransferase	アスパラギン酸アミノトランスフェラーゼ
	(glutamic oxaloacetic transaminase)	（グルタミン酸オキサロ酢酸トランスアミナーゼ）
AMI	acute myocardial infarction	急性心筋梗塞症
AML	acute myelocytic leukemia	急性骨髄性白血病
ARF	acute renal failure	急性腎不全
ASD	atrial septal defect	心房中隔不全
BBT	basal body temperature	基礎体温
BM	bowel movement	排便
BMD	bone mineral density	骨密度
BMI	body mass index	体格指数（＝体重／身長^2(kg/m^2)）
BMR	basal metabolic rate	基礎代謝率
BP	blood pressure	血圧
BS	breath sounds	呼吸音
	blood sugar	血糖
BSE	bovine spongiform encephalopathy	牛海綿状脳症，狂牛病
BW	body weight	体重
BWt	birth weight	出生時体重
CA	cancer, carcinoma	癌，腫
CAD	coronary artery disease	冠動脈不全
CBC	complete blood count	全血球計算
ChE	cholinesterase	コリンエステラーゼ
CHF	chronic heart failure	慢性心不全
CNS	central nervous system	中枢神経系
c/o	complains of	……を訴える
CRF	chronic renal failure	慢性腎不全

CT	cerebral tumor; coronary thrombosis	脳腫瘍；冠動脈血栓症
	computed tomography	コンピュータ断層撮影
Cx	cervix	頸部
CXR	chest X-ray	胸部 X 線撮影
DHF	Dengue hemorrhagic fever	デング出血熱
DM	diabetes mellitus	糖尿病
DU	duodenal ulcer	十二指腸潰瘍
ECG	electrocardiogram	心電図
ECT	emission computed tomography	放射型コンピュータ断層撮影
EEG	electroencephalogram	脳波（脳電図）
ENT	ear, nose and throat	耳，鼻，のど
ESWL	extracorporeal shock-wave lithotripsy	体外衝撃波結石
FBS	fasting blood sugar	空腹時血糖値
GA	general anesthetic	全身麻酔
GB	gallbladder	胆のう
GI	gastro-intestinal	胃・腸の
GU	gastric ulcer	胃潰瘍
Hb/Hgb	hemoglobin	ヘモグロビン
HBT	high blood pressure	高血圧
Hct (HCT)	hematocrit	ヘマトクリット（赤血球容積率）
HDL	high-density lipoprotein	善玉コレステロール（高密度リポタンパク質）
HepB (HB)	hepatitis B	B 型肝炎
HF	hay fever	花粉症，枯草熱
HIV	human immunodeficiency virus	ヒト免疫不全ウイルス
HP	history of present illness	現病歴
HR	heart rate	心拍数
IC	inspiratory capacity	深呼吸量
ICU	intensive care unit	集中治療部
iPS 細胞	induced pluripotent stem cell	誘導多能性幹細胞・人工万能幹細胞
IQ	intelligence quotient	知能指数
IV	intravenous	静脈内の
IVC	inferior vena cava	下大静脈
KUB	kidney, ureter and bladder	腎臓，尿管，膀胱
LDL	low-density lipoprotein	悪玉コレステロール（低密度コレステロール）
MCLS	mucocutaneous lymph node syndrome (Kawasaki disease)	［小児急性熱性］皮膚粘膜リンパ節症候群（川崎病）
MD	mental deficiency	精神遅滞
MI (MCI)	myocardial infarction	心筋梗塞

Appendix

MRI	magnetic resonance imaging	磁気共鳴画像法
MS	mitral stenosis; multiple sclerosis	僧帽弁狭窄症；多発性硬化症
MSW	medical social worker	医療ソーシャルワーカー
OA	on admission	入院中
OM	otitis media	中耳炎
OT	oculometric technician	視力検査士
P	pulse	脈拍
PD	Parkinson's disease	パーキンソン病
PET	positron emission tomography	陽電子放射型断層撮影法
PH	past history	既往歴
pH	power of potency	水素指数
pl.	plasma	血漿
PM	post mortem	検死，死体解剖
PMB	postmenopausal blooding	閉経後出血
PNS	peripheral nervous system	末梢神経系
PSW	psychiatric social worker	精神保健福祉士
p.o.	by mouth	経口で
R	right; respiration; red	右；呼吸；赤
RA	rheumatoid arthritis, red blood corpuscles	リューマチ様関節炎；赤血球
RBC	red blood cell count	赤血球数；赤血球
ref.	reference	参照・照合
RI	respiratory insufficiency	呼吸不全
RN	registered nurse	正看護師
S	single	独身
SARS	severe acute respiratory syndrome	重症急性呼吸器症候群
SMON	subacute myelo-optico-neuropathy	スモン病，亜急性脊髄視神経障害
SN	student nurse	看護学生
ST	speech therapist	言語療法士
T	temperature	体温
TB	tuberculosis	肺結核
Tcho	total cholesterol	総コレステロール
TPR	temperature, pulse, respiration	体温，脈拍，呼吸
UA	uric acid	尿酸
UTI	urinary tractinfection	尿路感染症
VC	vital capacity	肺活量
VSD	ventricular septal defect	心室中隔欠損症
W	widow/widower	やもめ（女性／男性）
WBC	white blood cell count; white blood corpuscles	白血球数；白血球
XR	X-ray	X線
YOB	year of birth	誕生年

注）略語のいくつかには，上記以外に複数の意味がある場合が多いので，用法に注意．

Prefix（接頭辞）

数を表す接頭辞

hemi-, semi-, demi-, (half)
hemiplegia 半身不随
semitendinous 半腱様の
demigod 半神半人

uni- （1）
uniceptor 単受体
unicuspid 一尖頭歯
unipara 1回経産婦
unisexual 単性の
unit 1個

bi- （2，2倍）
bicellular 2細胞性の
biceps 二頭筋
bichloride 二塩化物
bidermoma 二胚葉性混合腫瘍
bifurcation 分岐／分枝

di- （2倍）
dicephalus dipus 二頭二足二腕体
dibrachius
dichloride 二塩化物
dichromophilism 二染色性
dicoria 重複瞳孔
dicytosis 二種白血球増多症

semi- （半）
semiantigen 半抗原
semicoma 半昏睡
semilunar 半月状の
semiluxation 不全脱臼
semisupination 半上臥

tri- （3，3倍）
tricephalus 三頭体
triceps 三頭筋
tricuspid 三尖の，三尖弁の
trilobectomy 三肺葉切除
triplet 三胎，みつご

poly-, multi-, mult-, （多）
(many)polyhidrosis 多汗症
multiple fission 多分裂

Appendix

方向・位置の接頭辞

ex-, e-, ec-, ef-, es- exo- extra-, extro-	（外）	ante-, anti-, ant- pro- pre-	（前）
ad-, a-, af-, ag- al-, an-, ar-, as-, at-	（方向・到達）	post- re- retro-	（後）
ab-, abs-, a- dis-, dif-, di- de-, des- se-, sed- apo-, aph-	（分離）	super-, sur- extra- preter- ultra- hyper-	（上・超）
ambi- circum-, circu- peri-	（周囲）	de- sub-, suc-, suf-, sus-, sup- hypo-	（下）
juxta- para-	（近・傍）	in-, im-, il-, ir- en-, em- intro-, intra-, inter- endo-	（内）
per-, pel- trans- dia-	（貫通・横断）		

a-	（無，欠乏）	con-	（ともに，一緒に）
anidrosis	無汗症	concentration	濃縮，濃度
aphasia	失語症	congenital	先天性の
asexual	無性の	congestion	うっ血
asthenia	無力症	contact	接触
ab-	（離脱）	de-	（下方へ，～から，否定，欠如）
aberration	逸脱／異常		
abnormality	異常	deformation	奇形
abortion	流産	dehydration	脱水
abrasion	剥脱	delusion	妄想
		deposit	沈着物
amphi-	（両側，近傍，二重）	dia-	（～を通じて，横切って，間，隔離，完了）
amphiarthrosis	半関節		
amphibolia	疾患不定期		
amphidiarthrosis	複合関節	diagnosis	診断
amphinucleus	中心核	diaphragm	横隔膜
amphocyte	両染色性細胞	diarrhea	下痢
		diastalsis	波状蠕動
ante-	（時または場所の前）	dis-	（逆転，分離／重複）
ante cibum	食前	discharge	分泌
anteflexion	前屈	discission	切開
antenatal	出産前の	disease	病気，疾患
antepartum	分娩前の	disfunction	機能不全
antergy	拮抗作用		
ap/o-	（分離／誘導体）	en-	（中，内）
apocope	切断	encephalic	脳の
apophlegmatic	去痰剤	enclave	包入物
apositia	拒食症	encranial	頭蓋内の
apothanasia	延命	encyesis	子宮内妊娠
circum-	（周囲）	endo-	（内，内部）
circummaxillary	腋窩周囲の	endocrine	内分泌の
circumferentia	周径	endogenic	内部成長の，内因性の
circumnuclear	核周囲の		
circumstantiality	思考冗漫症	endometriosis	子宮内膜症
		endoscopy	内視鏡検査

Appendix

epi-, ep-	（上の，上方）	**infra-**	（下方，下部）
epidermis	表皮	infraduction	下転
epigastralgia	上腹部痛	infrapsychic	意識下の
epithelioma	上皮腫	infrascapular	肩甲骨下の
epizoon	外皮寄生虫	infraspinous	棘下の
ex-	（〜から離れた，〜なしの，外へ）	**intra-**	（内の）
exophthalmos	眼球突出	intracardiac	心臓内の
exotropia	外斜視	intracephalic	脳内の
exsanguinotransfusion	交換輸血法	intragenic	遺伝子内の
extraction	摘出	intraocular	眼球内の
extra-	（外側の，超えて，加えて）	**pan-**	（全，汎）
extra-anthropic	外的病因性の	panacea (panchrest)	万能薬
extracorporal (extrasomatic)	体外の	panagglutinins	汎凝集素
		pancreas	膵臓
extraligamentous	靱帯外の	pancytolysis	汎細胞崩壊
extrasystole	期外収縮		
extravasation	血管外遊出，浸潤		
hyper-	（上方，超，過剰）	**para-**	（側，向こうに，付属して）
hypercytosis	白血球増加症		
hyperemia	充血	paradentitis	歯周炎
hypertension	高血圧	paramenia	月経不順，月経困難
hypertrophy	肥大		
		paranoia	妄想症，偏執症
		parasympathitonia	副交感神経緊張症
hypo-	（下，以下，欠損）	**peri-**	（周囲の）
hypohepatia	肝機能低下	perimyositis	筋周囲炎
hypohydration	脱水症	periodontium	歯周組織
hypotension	低血圧	peritoneum	腹膜
hypothalamus	視床下部	peritonitis	腹膜炎

post-	(後の，次の，後ろの)	**supra-**	(上方に，上位に)
postadolescence	後思春期	supranormal	正常以上の
post cibum	食後	supraoptinum	最適上量
postclimacteric	更年期後の	suprarenalectomy	副腎摘出術
postembryonic	出生後の		
pre-	(あらかじめ，以前の，前の，……の前部にある)	**syn-**	(結合，共同)
		synchondrosis	軟骨結合
		syndrome	症候群
		synesthesia	共感覚
precancer	前癌状態	synostosis	骨結合
premature	早熟，早発		
predisposition	素質，体質		
presenile	初老期の，初老性の		
retr/o-	(後方，逆行)	**trans-**	(〜を通して，〜を横切って)
retrocatheterism	逆行カテーテル法	transference	転移
retroflexion	後屈	transfusion	輸血
retrostalsis	逆蠕動	transgenic	トランスジェニック
retroversion	後反	translocation	転位，転置
sub-	(下，下位，副，亜)	**ultra-**	(過剰，超過)
subconsciousness	潜在意識	ultracentrifuge	超遠心分離器
subcutaneous	皮下の	ultrasonogram	超音波検査図
subfertility	低受精率	ultrastructure	超微細構造
submania	軽躁病，躁病	ultraviolet	紫外線
super-	(上，過剰)		
superalimentation (supernutrition)	栄養過多		
superficial	表面の		
superinfection	重複感染		
supersecretion	過分泌		

Appendix

Suffix（疾患とかかわる接尾辞）

-ia	（病名・症状・種の生物現象）	-phobia	[Gk. *phobos* ＋ -ia]
analgesia	無痛覚	hydrophobia	恐水病／狂犬病
aphasia	失語症	necrophobia	死亡恐怖／死体恐怖
bulimia	大食		
diphtheria	ジフテリア	schoolphobia	登校拒否症
hysteria	ヒステリー	xenophobia	他人恐怖症
ophthalmia	眼炎		
urticaria	じんま疹		

以下語根＋-ia で接尾辞扱い

-algia	（痛む状態）[Gk. *algos* ＋ -ia]	-gen, -gene	（〜を生ずるもの，〜から生じたもの）
cardialgia	心臓痛		
dentalgia	歯痛	allergen	アレルゲン
gasteralgia	胃痛	carcinogen	発癌物質
otalgia	耳痛	oxygen	酸素
		pathogen	病原体

-dynia	[Gk. *dyn-* ＋ -ia]	-itis	（語幹の示す部位の炎症）
cardiodynia	心臓痛		
dorsodynia	背痛	bronchitis	気管支炎
gastrodynia	胃痛	hepatitis	肝炎
otodynia	耳痛	otitis media	中耳炎

注）連結形には -dynia，語根には -algia をつける．

		rheumatoid arthritis	リューマチ様関節炎
		stomatitis	口内炎

-mania	[Gk. *mani* ＋ -ia]	-osis	（疾患・病的経過）
logomania	多弁症	arteriosclerosis	動脈硬化
megalomania	誇大妄想	liver cirrhosis	肝硬変
phagomania	貪食症	nephrelcosis	腎臓潰瘍
pseudomania	偽精神症	neurosis	ノイローゼ／神経症
		pollenosis	花粉症

-pathy	[Gk. *pathos* + -y]	**-ectomy**	（切除術）ec-（外へ）＋ -tomy（切開術）
adenopathy	腺症		
hepatic encephalopathy	肝性脳症	adenoidectomy	アデノイド切除術
osteopathy	骨疾患		
syphilopathy	梅毒	cholecystectomy	胆のう切除術
		duodenectomy	十二指腸切除術
		gastrectomy	胃切除術
		keratectomy	角膜切除術
		mammectomy	乳房切除術
		myomectomy	筋腫切除術
		oophorectomy	卵巣切除術
		polypectomy	ポリープ切除術
-oma	（腫瘍・腫瘤）	**-o/stomy**	（造屡術／吻合術）
adenoma	腺腫	appendicocecostomy	虫垂結腸吻合術
carcinoma	癌腫	cholangio-enterostomy	胆管腸管吻合術
lymphoma	リンパ腫	enteroenterostomy	腸腸吻合術
oophoroma	卵巣腫	esophagoduodenostomy	食道十二指腸吻合術
sarcoma	肉腫		
		gastroduodenostomy	胃十二指腸吻合術
		hepatocholangio-cystoduodenostomy	肝内胆管十二指腸吻合術
		ileocolostomy	回結腸吻合術
		ovariostomy	卵巣吻合術
		venovenostomy	静脈静脈吻合術
		vesicostomy	膀胱造屡術
-oid	（語幹についてそれに類似しているものを表す）	**-o/tomy**	（切開・切開術）
		anatomy	解剖
lipoid	類脂	antiotomy	扁桃切開術
mucoid	粘液様の	chondrotomy	軟骨切開術
paranoid	偏執病様の	craniotomy	頭蓋切開術
thyroid	甲状腺の	herniotomy	ヘルニア切開術
		necrotomy	死体解剖
		thoracotomy	開胸術

-logy, -logist については medical staff の項参照

Appendix

Combining forms and medical terms（連結形）

（o は連結母音）

abdomin/o-	（腹部）	**arteri/o-**	（動脈）
abdominocentesis	腹部穿刺	arterionecrosis	動脈壊死
abdominocystic	腹胆嚢の	arteriomalacia	——軟化症
abdominoscopy	腹腔鏡検査	arteriosclerosis	——硬化症
abdominal cavity	腹腔	arteriospasm	——痙攣
acr/o-	（四肢，先端，頂，極端）	**bi/o-**	（生命・生活）
acroagnosis	四肢感覚失認症	biomicroscopy	生体顕微鏡検査
acrocephalopolysyndactyly	尖頭多指癒合症	bionecrosis	類壊死
acrocyanosis	先端チアノーゼ	biopsy	生検
acromegaly	先端巨大症	biotomy	生体解剖
aden/o-	（腺）	**-blast, blast/o-**	（芽細胞）
adenochondrosarcoma	腺軟骨肉腫	angioblast	脈管胚葉
adenocyte	腺細胞	myoblast	筋芽細胞
adenofibrosis	腺繊維症	spermatoblast	精芽細胞
adenohypersthenia	腺分泌機能亢進	blastoderm	胞胚葉
angi/o-	（血管）	**blephar/o-**	（眼瞼，眼毛）
angioedema	血管浮腫	blepharoconjunctivitis	——結膜炎
angiohemaphilia	血管血友病	blepharoplasty	——形成術
angiolymphoma	血管リンパ腫	blepharorrhaphy	——縫合術
angiospasm	血管痙攣	blepharosphincterectomy	——括約筋切除
ankyl/o-	（曲がった）	**brachy-**	（短い）
ankylocheilia	口唇拘着症	brachyesophagus	食道短縮
ankyloglossia	舌小帯短縮症	brachymetatarsia	短中足症
ankylotia	外耳道孔閉鎖	brachymetropia	近視
ankylurethria	尿道狭窄	brachyphalangia	短指節症
arthr/o-	（関節）	**brady-**	（遅い）
arthralgia	関節痛	bradycardia	徐脈
arthrodesis	関節固定術	bradyesthesia	知覚遅鈍
arthroheumatism	関節リウマチ	bradylalia	言語緩慢，遅語
arthritis	関節炎	bradypnea	呼吸緩徐

bronch/o-	(気管支)	**cheil/o-**	(唇，唇の縁)
bronchiectasis	気管支拡張症	cheilognathopalatoschisis	唇顎口蓋裂
bronchopneumonia	気管支肺炎	cheiloncus	口唇の腫瘍
bronchospasm	気管支痙攣	cheiloschisis	口唇裂，兎唇
bronchostaxis	気管支壁出血	cheilostomatoplasty	唇口腔形成術
carcin/o-	(癌)	**chem/o-, chemi-**	(化学・化学薬品)
carcinogenesis	発癌		
carcinoma	癌腫	cheminosis	化学因性疾患
carcinomelcosis	悪性潰瘍	chemobiotic	化学抗生剤
carcinomatophobia	発癌恐怖症	chemodectoma	化学感受体腫
		chemotherapy	化学療法
cardi/o-	(心臓)	**chol-, chole-, chol/o-**	(胆汁)
cardialgia	胸やけ	cholecystitis	胆嚢炎
cardiasthma	心臓性喘息	cholelithotripsy	胆石破砕術
cardiodynia	心臓痛	cholemesis	胆汁嘔吐症
cardiovalvulitis	心臓弁膜炎	cholemia	胆血症
cephal/o-	(頭)	**chondr/o-**	(軟骨)
cephalocentesis	頭蓋穿刺	chondrification	軟骨化，軟骨形成
cephalomeningitis	脳膜炎		
cephalothoracopagus	頭胸結合体	chondrodysplasia	軟骨形成不全
histamine cephalagia	ヒスタミン頭痛症	chondrodystrophia	軟骨形成異常
		chondrosarcoma	軟骨肉腫
cerebr/o-	(脳)	**col/o-**	(結腸)
cerebromalacia	脳軟化症	colodyspepsia	結腸性消化不良症
cerebrospinal meningitis	脳脊髄膜炎		
cerebropsychosis	脳性精神症	colonoscopy	結腸内視鏡
cerebrosclerosis	脳硬化症	coloptosis	結腸下垂症
		colopuncture	結腸穿刺
cervic/o-	(頸部)	**colp/o-**	(膣)
cervicitis	子宮頸炎	colpopolypus	膣ポリープ
cervicocolpitis	子宮頸管膣炎	colporrhaphy	膣縫合術
cervicovaginitis	子宮頸膣炎	colporrhexis	膣裂傷
cervicobrachialgia	頸腕痛	colpospasm	膣痙
cervicoplasty	頸形成術	colpostenosis	膣狭窄

Appendix

crani/o-	(頭蓋)(とうがい)	**dipl/o-**	(二重, 双, 二倍, 二度)
craniomalacia	頭蓋軟化症	diplegia	両側麻痺
craniopharyngioma	頭蓋咽頭腫	diplobacterium	双桿菌
craniostenosis	狭頭症	diplococcus	双球菌
craniotrypesis	開頭術	diplopia	二重視
cyst/o-	(袋・嚢)	**duoden/o-**	(十二指腸)
cystirrhea	膀胱カタル	duodenocholangeitis	十二指腸総胆管炎
cystolithaiasis	膀胱結石症		
cystomyxoadenoma	嚢腫様筋腺腫	duodenogram	十二指腸X線像
cystopyelonephritis	膀胱腎盂腎炎	duodenolysis	十二指腸剝離術
		duodenoscopy	十二指腸鏡検査法
cyt/o-	(細胞)	**encephal/o-**	(脳)
cytodieresis	細胞分裂	encephalitogen	脳炎誘発物質
cytogenesis	細胞発生	encephaloma	脳腫瘤
cytoplasm	細胞形質	encephalomalacia	脳軟化症
cytostasis	細胞性塞	encephalonarcosis	脳性昏迷
		encephalosepsis	脳壊疽
dactyl/o-	(通常手指・時折足指)	**enter/o-**	(腸)
dactylium	合指症	enterproctia	人工肛門
dactylogram	指紋	enteroscope	腸鏡
dactylolysis	指切断	enterosite	腸内寄生虫
dactylospasm	指痙攣	enterostasis	腸閉塞
dent/o-	(歯)	**eu-**	(良い, 容易, 健康)
dentifrice	歯みがき剤		
dentition	歯列・生歯	europelstalsis	正常蠕動
dentode	デントード	euphoria	多幸症
denture	義歯	eutocia	正常分娩
		eutrophia	栄養良好
dermat/o-	(皮膚)	**fibr/o-**	(線維)
atopic dermatitis	アトピー性皮膚炎	cystic fibrosis	嚢胞性線維症
		fibrocarcinoma	線維癌腫
dermatocandidiasis	皮膚カンジダ症	fibrocartilage	線維軟骨
dermatosis	皮膚病	fibromyositis	線維筋炎
roentgen-ray dermatitis	X線皮膚炎		

gastr/o-	（胃）	**gynec/o-, gynaec/o,**	（女性）
gastrectasia	胃拡張	gyn-, gyne-, gyno-	
gastroenteroptosis	胃腸下垂症	gynecoid obesity	女性様肥満
gastrorrhea	胃液分泌過多症	gynopathy	婦人病
gastroscope	胃鏡	gynephobia	女性恐怖症
		gynogenesis	雌核発生
gen/o-	（遺伝子，因子）	**hem/o-, haem/o, hema-, haema-, hemat/**	（血液）
biogenesis	生物発生		
generation	生殖行動／世代／発生	hemacyte (hemocyte, hematocyte)	血球
genetic map	遺伝子地図	hemolysis	溶血
X-linked gene	X染色体遺伝子	hematuria	血尿
		hemodialyzer	血液透析器
genit/o-	（生殖器）	**hepat/o-**	（肝臓）
genitalia	生殖器	heptargia	肝機能不全
genitoinfectiouos	性病の	hepatocirrhosis	肝硬変
genitoplasty	生殖器形成術	hepatomegaly	肝肥大
genitourinary	尿生殖器	hepatoperitonitis	肝部腹膜炎
gingiv/o-	（歯肉）	**hydr/o-**	（水／水素）
gingivectomy	歯肉切除術	hydroa	水疱症
gingivoglossitis	歯肉舌炎	hydroblepharon	眼瞼浮腫
gingivostomatitis	歯肉口内炎	hydrodipsia	水分渇望
herpetic gingivitis	ヘルペス性歯肉炎	hydrotherapy	水治療法
gloss/o-	（舌）	**hyster/o-**	（子宮／ヒステリー）
glossocoma	舌収縮		
glossopalatinus	舌口蓋筋	hysteroepilepsy	ヒステリー性てんかん
glossopyrosis	舌灼熱感		
hypoglossal nerve	舌下神経	hysteromyoma	子宮筋腫
		hysteroptosis	子宮下垂
		hysterovaginoenterocele	子宮・膣・腸ヘルニア
glyc/o-	（糖）	**kinesi/o-, kine-**	（運動）
glycemia	血糖症	bradykinesia	運動緩慢
glycogen	グリコーゲン	kinesitherapy	筋運動療法
glycolipid	糖脂質	kenesia	運動症・乗物酔
glycopolyuria	糖尿病性多尿	kinetochore	動原体
glycorrhachia	糖性脳脊髄液症		

Appendix

lact/o-	(乳)	**lith/o-**	(石, 結石)
lactase	ラクターゼ(乳酸分解酵素)	litholysis	結石溶解
		lithomyl	膀胱結石粉砕器
lacteal	乳糜リンパ管	lithonephria	腎結石症
lactivorous	哺乳の	lithuria	尿酸(塩)尿(症)
lapar/o-	(腹部/側腹部)	**lob/o-**	(葉)
laparogastroscopy	腹式胃鏡検査法	lobitis	肺葉炎
laparohysterosalpingo-oophorectomy	腹式卵管卵巣摘除術	lobe of lung	肺葉
		lobule	小葉
laparorrhagy	腹壁縫合術	lobus	葉
laparotomy	開腹術		
laryng/o-	(喉頭)	**log/o-**	(言語)
laryngitis	喉頭炎	logoneurosis	神経性言語障害
laryngomalacia	喉頭軟化症	logorrhea	病的多弁症
laryngoparalysis (laryngoplegia)	喉頭麻痺	logospasm	痙攣性発語
laryngorrhagia	喉頭出血		
leuc/o-, leuk/o-	(白い)	**lymph/o-**	(リンパ)
leucocytosis	白血球増多症	lymphadenhypertrophy	リンパ節肥大
leukemia	白血病	lymphadenomatosis	リンパ節腫症
leukorrhea	白帯下/こしけ	lymphatolysis	リンパ組織崩壊
leukothrombopenia	白血球血小板減少症	lymphoma	リンパ腫
lip/o-	(脂肪)	**-o/lysis**	(溶解/分解)
liparodyspnea	肥満者呼吸困難	hemolysis	溶血
lipase	リパーゼ(脂肪分解酵素)	lipolysis	脂肪分解
		nephrolysis	腎物質溶解
lipophagia	脂肪沈着症	spermatolysis	精子溶解/精子破壊
lipophagy	脂肪吸収		

macr/o-	（巨大なこと／異常な大きさ，長さ）	**micr/o-**	（微少／単位 10^{-6}）
macrocyte	大赤血球	micromyelolymphocyte	小骨髄芽（リンパ）球
macrolide	マクロライド［抗生物質］	microelements	微量元素
macrostomia	巨口症	microtransfusion	微量輸血
macula	汚点／斑点／肥厚	microvilli	微繊毛
malac/o-	（異常な軟化状態を表す）	**mit/o-**	（糸状）
arteriomalacia	動脈軟化症	mitochondria	ミトコンドリア／糸球体
malactic	皮膚軟化剤	mitosis	有糸分裂
nephromalacia	腎軟化症	mitosome	ミトソーム
osteomalacia	骨軟化症		
megal/o-, megas, megale-	（巨大）	**mon/o-**	（1つ／単一）
megaloblast	巨大赤芽球	monaxon	単軸索ニューロン
megalocardia	心臓肥大	monoanesthesia	局所麻酔
megaloenteron	腸拡張症	monocular	単眼性の
megalothymus	胸腺肥大	mononeuritis	単神経炎
mening/o-	（脳・脊髄をおおう膜）	**muc/o-**	（粘液）
meningiomatosis	髄膜腺腫	mucinuria	粘液尿
meningocele	髄膜瘤，髄膜ヘルニア	mucocolitis	粘液性結腸炎
meningomyelitis	髄膜脊髄炎	mucoenteritis	小腸粘膜炎
meningorrhea	髄膜内出血	mucopus	膿様粘液
men/o-	（月経）	**multi-**	（多数，多量）
amenorrhea	無月経	multicellular	多細胞の
dysmenorrhea	月経困難症	multi-infection	多感染
menarche	初潮	multipara	経産婦
menopause	閉経（期）	multisentivity	多感受性

Appendix

myc/o-, mycet-	(真菌)	**nephr/o-**	(腎)
mycodermatitis	真菌皮膚炎	nephratonia	腎無力症
mycophagy	菌食	nephropyelography	腎・腎盂造影法
mycoplasma	マイコプラズマ	nephrosclerosis	腎硬化症
mycotoxin	かび中毒／真菌毒	nephrosis	腎症／ネフローゼ
myel/o-	(髄)	**neur/o-**	(神経)
myelocystomeningocele	脊髄囊髄膜瘤	neurodynia	神経痛
myeloma	骨髄腫	neuroparalysis	神経麻痺
myeloplegia	脊髄麻痺	neuropsychosis	神経精神病
myeloscintigram	脊髄シンチグラム	neurosis	神経症／ノイローゼ
my/o-	(筋)	**nyct/o-**	(夜)
myocardiopathy	心筋障害	nyctophilia	暗夜嗜好症
myodynamometer	筋力計	nyctophobia	くらやみ恐怖
myodystrophia	筋ジストロフィー	nyctophonia	夜間発声
myopericarditis	心筋心囊炎	nycturia	夜間頻尿
narc/o-	(昏迷, 昏迷状態)	**o/o-**	(卵／卵子)
narcoanalysis	麻酔分析	oocyesis	卵巣妊娠
narcoanesthesia	昏迷麻酔	oocyte	卵母細胞
narcosis	麻酔法	ookinesis	卵子分裂
narcotism	麻酔／麻酔嗜癖	oosperm	受精卵
necr/o-	(死, 死体, 死細胞)	**oophor/o-**	(卵巣)
necremia	敗血症	oophoroma	卵巣腫
necrocytosis	細胞壊死	oophoropathy	卵巣疾患
necroscopy	剖検, 検死	oophorosalpingitis	卵巣卵管炎
necrosis	壊死	oophorrhagia	卵巣過剰出血
ne/o-	(新しい)	**ophthalm/o-**	(眼)
neogenesis	新生	ophthalmocopia	眼精疲労
neolallism	新語多発症	ophthalmoscope	検眼鏡
neomembrane	偽膜	ophthalmotonometry	眼圧測定
neonatal	新生児期		

orchid/o-, orchi/o	（精巣／睾丸）	**ov/o-, ovi-**	（卵／卵子）
orchiocele	睾丸ヘルニア	ovocyte	卵母細胞
orchioncus	睾丸腫瘍	ovogenesis	卵子発生
orchioscirrhus	睾丸硬化症	ovulation	排卵
orchis	精巣，睾丸	ovum	卵／卵子
orth/o-	（まっすぐな／正常な）	**path/o-**	（疾患）
orthodontia	歯科矯正学	pathoclisis	特異的過敏症
orthophoria	眼球正位	patholysis	疾病消失
orthopia	斜視予防	pathomimesis	仮病
orthotics	矯正学	pathoneurosis	病的神経症
osm/o-	（におい）	**ped/o-**	（足／小児）
osmodysphoria	臭気嫌悪性	pedodontics	小児歯科
osmoreceptor	浸透圧受容器	pedometer	歩数計
osmoscope	嗅覚器	pedopathy	足疾患
osmosis	浸透	pedunculotomy	脳脚切開
oste/o-	（骨）	**phag/o-**	（食）
osteoarthropathy	骨関節症	phagocyte	食細胞
osteochondritis	骨軟骨症	phagocytosis	食作用
osteodystrophy	骨ジストロフィー（骨形成異常）	phagophobia	食事恐怖症
		phagotherapy	食事療法
osteoporosis	骨粗鬆症		
ot/o-	（耳）	**phleb/o-**	（静脈）
otitis media	中耳炎	phleboclysis	静脈注射
otorrhea	耳漏	phlebonarcosis	静脈内麻酔法
otosis	誤聴／錯聴	phlebostasia	静脈血うっ滞
		phlebothrombosis	静脈血栓症
ovari/o-	（卵巣）	**phon/o-**	（音，声）
ovariocyesis	卵巣妊娠	phonacoscope	聴打診器
ovariohysterectomy	卵巣子宮切除術	phoniatrician	音声治療士
ovariorrhexis	卵巣破裂	phonocardiograph	心音計
ovarium	卵巣	phonoreception	音覚認知

Appendix

phren/o-	（横隔膜／精神）	**prot/o-**	（最初）
phrenetic	躁病患者	protoplasia	原形成
phrenopericarditis	横隔膜心膜炎	protoplasm	原形質
phrenospasm	横隔膜痙攣	prototype	原型
schizophrenia	統合失調症	protozoan	原生動物
pleur/o-	（胸膜／側胸部／肋骨）	**pseud/o-**	（偽）
pleuritis	胸膜炎	pseudoasthma	偽性喘息
pleuroclysis	胸膜腔洗浄	pseudocyesis	偽妊娠
pleurorrhea	胸腔漏	pseudoesthesia	幻感覚
		pseudogout	偽性痛風
-pnea	（呼吸）	**psych/o-**	（精神／心）
apnea	無呼吸	psychoanalysis	精神分析
bradypnea	呼吸緩除	psychogenesis	精神作用
dyspnea	呼吸困難	psychosis	精神病
tachypnea	頻呼吸	psychology	心理学
pneum/o-	（肺）	**-ptosis**	（下垂）
pneumocentesis	肺穿刺	blepharoptosis	眼瞼下垂
pneumohemothorax	気血胸	coloptosis	結腸下垂
pneumonia	肺炎	hysteroptosis	子宮下垂
pneumopyothorax	膿気胸	nephroptosis	腎下垂
poly-	（多数／多量）	**pyel/o-**	（腎盂）
polyneuritis	多発性神経炎	pyelitis	腎盂炎
polyphagia	多食症	pyelocystitis	腎盂膀胱炎
polypharmacy	多剤投与	pyelonephritis	腎盂腎炎
polyuria	多尿症	pyelostomy	腎盂造瘻術
proct/o-	（直腸）	**py/o-**	（膿）
proctoclysis	直腸灌注	pyocele	膿瘤
proctoparalysis	肛門括約筋麻痺	pyodermatits	化膿性皮膚炎
proctoptosis	脱肛	pyorrhea	膿漏
proctostomy	人工肛門形成	pyothorax	膿胸

pyr/o-	(火，熱，[化学]加熱によって生じる)	**ser/o-**	(漿液／血清)
pyrolysis	熱分解	seroculture	血清培養
pyromania	放火癖	serositis	漿膜炎
pyrophobia	恐火症	serotherapy	血清療法
pyrosis	胸やけ	serotype	血清型
rachi/o-	(脊柱)	**sial/o-**	(唾液)
rachiocentesis	脊椎穿刺	sialoadenectomy	唾液腺切除(術)
rachiotome	脊椎切断器	sialagogue	催唾液薬
rachioplegia	脊髄麻痺	sialorrhea	唾液分泌
rachisensibility	脊椎麻酔過敏症	sialoschesis	唾液分泌抑制
radi/o-	(放射線)	**somat/o-**	(身体／躯幹)
radiocarcinogenesis	放射線発癌	somatoceptor	体感受容器
radiodensity	放射線濃度	somatogenesitis	体発達
radiodiagnosis	X 線診断法	somatometry	身体測定
radioimmunity	放射線免疫	somatotonia	身体緊張型
sarco/o-	(肉)	**spermat/o-, sperm/o-**	(種：特に男性の生殖要素)
sarcoidosis	類肉腫症		
sarcolemma	筋線維膜	spermatocystitis	精嚢炎
sarcoma	肉腫	spermatosome,	精子
sarcosis	筋肉瘤腫	spermatozoon	
		spermatoblast	精子細胞
		spermoplasm	精細胞形質
scler/o-	(硬い)	**sphygm/o-**	(脈拍)
scleradenitis	硬性リンパ節炎	sphygmobolometry	脈圧力測定法
sclerema	強膜硬化症	sphygmocardiogram	脈拍心拍曲線
scleroderma	強皮症	sphygmometer	血圧測定
sclerosis	硬化症	sphygmopalpation	脈拍触診
scot/o-	(暗)	**staphyl/o-**	(口蓋垂／ブドウ球菌)
scotoma	(視野)暗点		
scotophilia	暗所嗜好症	staphylocide	殺ブドウ球菌剤
scotophobia	——恐怖症	staphylococosis	ブドウ球菌症
scotopia	——視	staphylococcus	ブドウ球菌
		staphyloptosis	口蓋垂下垂症

Appendix

stern/o-	（胸骨）	**thyr/o-**	（甲状腺）
sternodynia	胸骨痛	thyrocarditis	甲状腺性心炎
sternotomy	胸骨切開	thyroiditis	甲状腺炎
sternotrypesis	胸骨穿孔術	thyromegaly	甲状腺肥大
sternum	胸骨	thyroprivia	甲状腺欠損
stomat/o-	（口／子宮）	**tox/o-**	（毒素／毒）
stomatitis	口内炎	antitoxin	抗毒素
stomatodysodia	口臭	toxin	毒素／トキシン
stomatorrhagia	口内出血	toxoid	類毒素
stomatotomy	子宮口切開術	toxinosis	中毒症
therm/o-	（熱）	**troph/o-**	（食物／栄養）
thermoanesthesia	温覚消失	trophoblastoma	栄養膜
thermohypesthesia	温覚過敏	trophoneurosis	栄養神経症
thermolysis	加熱分解	trophopathia	栄養障害
thermometer	温度計	trophotherapy	栄養療法
thorac/o-	（胸）	**viscero-**	（腹部）
thoracentesis	胸腔穿刺	visceralgia	内臓痛
thoracoceloschisis	胸腹壁破裂	viscerography	内臓造影法
thoracoscope	胸腔鏡／聴診器	visceroptosis	内臓下垂症
thoracostenosis	胸郭狭窄	viscerotome	内臓切除刀
thromb/o-	（凝血塊／血栓）		
thrombocyte	血小板		
thromboembolism	血餅塞形成		
thrombolymphangitis	血栓性リンパ管炎		
thrombophlebitis	血栓静脈炎		

色に関する連結形

chlor/o- （緑）
chlorenchyma　　　葉緑組織
chlorolymphosarcoma　緑色リンパ肉腫
chloroma　　　　　緑色骨髄腫
chlorophyl　　　　クロロフィル／
　　　　　　　　　葉緑素
chlorosarcoma　　　緑色肉腫

cyan/o- （青い）
autotoxic cyanosis　自家中毒性チア
　　　　　　　　　ノーゼ
cyanogen　　　　　シアン
cyanopia　　　　　青視症
cyanopsin　　　　シアノプシン
cyanosis　　　　　チアノーゼ

erythr/o- （赤い）
erythrocyte　　　　赤血球
erythrocytolysis　　溶血
erythrocyturia　　　血尿症
erythrokeratodermia　紅斑角皮症
erythropenia　　　 赤血球減少

leuk/o-, leuc/o- （白い）
leukemia　　　　　白血病
leukencephalitis　　脳白質炎
leukopenia　　　　白血球減少症
leukocytosis　　　 白血球増加症
leukorrhea　　　　白帯下，こしけ
leukotomy　　　　白質切除術

melan/o- （黒い）
melancholia　　　　メランコリー／
　　　　　　　　　うつ病
melanin　　　　　　メラニン
melanoblastoma　　　黒色芽腫
melanoma　　　　　黒色腫
melena　　　　　　メレナ／黒色便

xanth/o- （黄色い）
xanthemia　　　　　黄色血症
xanthocyte　　　　黄色細胞
xanthogranuloma　　黄色肉芽腫
xanthosarcoma　　　黄色肉腫
xanthosis　　　　　黄変

著者紹介

清水　雅子
 1982年 岡山大学大学院教育学研究科英語教育専攻修士課程修了
    元 川崎医療福祉大学医療福祉学部／大学院医療福祉研究科 教授，
    元 北里大学一般教育部 非常勤講師
 著　書 「医療技術者のための医学英語入門」(1991)，「病気の英語入門」(1994)，「はじめての栄養英語」(2007)，「はじめての臨床栄養英語」(2013，共著)，以上講談社．「ドーランド図説医学大辞典第28版」(1997，分担執筆)，以上廣川書店．「福祉・介護学生のための総合英語」(2007)，以上南雲堂．「リハビリテーションの基礎英語改訂第2版」(2016)，「リハビリテーション英語の基本用語と表現」(2015)，以上メジカルビュー社．「PT・OT・STのための国際学会はじめの一歩」(2014)，以上三輪書店．

NDC 491 213 p 21cm

医療従事者のための医学英語入門

2011年3月10日 第 1 刷発行
2025年7月18日 第16刷発行

著　者	清水雅子
発行者	篠木和久
発行所	株式会社　講談社

KODANSHA

〒112-8001　東京都文京区音羽2-12-21
  販売　(03) 5395-5817
  業務　(03) 5395-3615

編　集 株式会社　講談社サイエンティフィク
   代表　堀越俊一
   〒162-0825　東京都新宿区神楽坂2-14　ノービィビル
    編集　(03) 3235-3701

印刷所 株式会社双文社印刷・半七写真印刷工業株式会社
製本所 株式会社国宝社

落丁本・乱丁本は，購入書店名を明記のうえ，講談社業務宛にお送り下さい．送料小社負担にてお取り替えします．なお，この本の内容についてのお問い合わせは講談社サイエンティフィク宛にお願いいたします．定価はカバーに表示してあります．

©Masako Shimizu, 2011

本書のコピー，スキャン，デジタル化等の無断複製は著作権法上での例外を除き禁じられています．本書を代行業者等の第三者に依頼してスキャンやデジタル化することはたとえ個人や家庭内の利用でも著作権法違反です．

Printed in Japan
ISBN 978-4-06-155615-7

講談社の自然科学書

はじめての栄養英語
清水 雅子・著
B5・108頁・定価1,980円（税込）
やさしい英文で初学者でも栄養英語に親しめるよう工夫されたテキスト。栄養素、代謝、解剖生理、消化吸収、食品添加物、食物アレルギーなどを、やさしく短い英文でとりあげた。

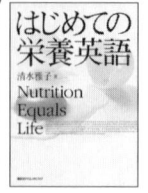

やさしい英語ニュースで学ぶ 現代社会と健康
田中芳文・編著
B5・109頁・定価2,640円（税込）
医療・福祉・栄養系など、健康とふかくかかわる学生のための教科書。とくに現代社会とのかかわりを意識させる英語ニュースをピックアップ。

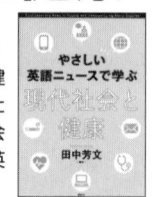

はじめての臨床栄養英語
清水 雅子／J.パトリック バロン・著
B5・121頁・定価2,530円（税込）
栄養管理を必要とする疾患を中心に、平易な英文で、組織・器官の名称、病気の概要、診断基準、食事療法、薬物療法を学ぶこれまでにない教科書。病院臨地実習やゼミで必須となる基本英語を集約。大学院受験にも役立つ。

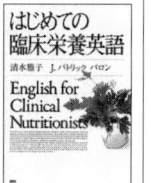

英文ニュースで学ぶ 健康とライフスタイル
田中芳文・編著
B5・109頁・定価2,860円（税込）
医療や健康の話題を扱ったニュース記事で英語リーディング能力をレベルアップ！一般人向けの記事だから、出てくる用語は一般常識レベルで、文章も読みやすい。

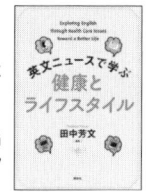

Let's Study English! Health and Nutrition 英語で読む健康と栄養
横尾 信男・編著
A5・94頁・定価1,650円（税込）
栄養系学生のための教養課程英語テキスト。健康な食生活に必要な知識（栄養素やその摂取法、病気にならない食生活・エクササイズ、酒やタバコの害、食中毒、ストレス解消など）を幅広く学べるよう編集。

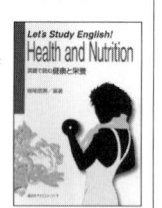

アカデミック・フレーズバンク
そのまま使える！構文200・文例1900
ジョン・モーリー・著／高橋さきの・訳／国枝哲夫・監修
B5変・272頁・定価2,750円（税込）
世界中の研究者に愛用されているウェブサイト「Academic Phrasebank」の邦訳書がついに登場。これが、英語論文によく使う表現文例集の決定版。日本語訳付きは便利でやっぱり安心。そのまま使える！ずっと使える！

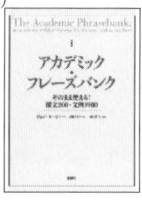

ネイティブが教える 日本人研究者のための 論文の書き方・アクセプト術
エイドリアン・ウォールワーク・著 前平謙二／笠川梢・訳
A5・512頁・定価4,180円（税込）
これほど網羅的で深い示唆を与えてくれる指南書はほかにない！ネイティブの思考・語感で、ワンランク上の論文に！そのまま使える論文英語表現を580例も掲載！

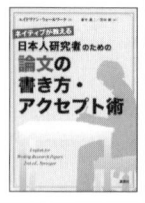

ネイティブが教える 日本人研究者のための 論文英語表現術 文法・語法・言い回し
エイドリアン・ウォールワーク・著 前平謙二／笠川梢・訳
A5・320頁・定価3,080円（税込）
冠詞の使い分けから時制、仮定法、接続詞の使い方、語順のポイントに至るまで、ネイティブらしい自然な言い回しのコツを225項目掲載。

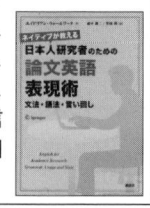

表示価格は税込です。

「2025年6月20日現在」

講談社サイエンティフィク　https://www.kspub.co.jp/